Answers
for the

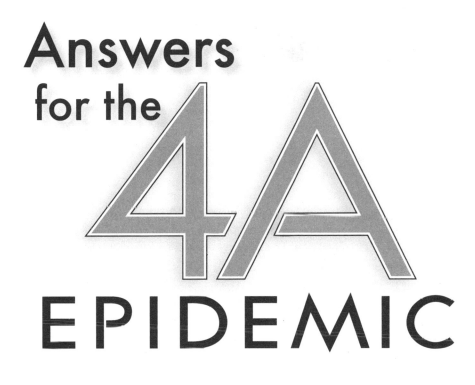

4A
EPIDEMIC

Joseph A. Cannizzaro, MD

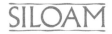

SILOAM

Most CHARISMA HOUSE BOOK GROUP products are available at special quantity discounts for bulk purchase for sales promotions, premiums, fund-raising, and educational needs. For details, write Charisma House Book Group, 600 Rinehart Road, Lake Mary, Florida 32746, or telephone (407) 333-0600.

ANSWERS FOR THE 4-A EPIDEMIC by Joseph A. Cannizzaro, MD
Published by Siloam
Charisma Media/Charisma House Book Group
600 Rinehart Road
Lake Mary, Florida 32746
www.charismahouse.com

Cover design by Ashley Willsey
Design Director: Bill Johnson

Visit the author's websites at www.AccordoHealth.com, www.JPCAC.com, and www .PediatriciansCareUnit.com.

Library of Congress Cataloging-in-Publication Data:
An application to register this book for cataloging has been submitted to the Library of Congress.
International Standard Book Number: 978-1-61638-484-5
E-book ISBN: 978-1-61638-702-0

This book contains the opinions and ideas of its author. It is solely for informational and educational purposes and should not be regarded as a substitute for professional medical treatment. The nature of your body's health condition is complex and unique. Therefore you should consult a health professional before you begin any new exercise, nutrition, or supplementation program or if you have questions about your health. Neither the author nor the publisher shall be liable or responsible for any loss or damage allegedly arising from any information or suggestion in this book.

People and names in this book are composites created by the author from his experiences as a medical doctor. Names and details of their stories have been changed, and any similarity between the names and stories of individuals described in this book to individuals known to readers is purely coincidental.

The statements in this book about consumable products or food have not been evaluated by the Food and Drug Administration. The publisher is not responsible

While the author has made every effort to provide accurate telephone numbers and Internet addresses at the time of publication, neither the publisher nor the author assumes any responsibility for errors or for changes that occur after publication.

First edition
12 13 14 15 16 — 987654321
Printed in the United States of America

DEDICATION

I dedicate this book to the following: my father, Mr. P. Cannizzaro, who led me on an unrelenting quest for wisdom, and to my mother, Mrs. K. Cannizzaro, whose unconditional love and deep compassion for all those in need were the inspiration to begin my journey in medicine; my beautiful spouse, Carol Ann, who has made the last forty-three years of my life the most wonderful any husband could imagine; and my three sons, Joe Jr., Tom, and Marc, who have made my life as a father very meaningful.

I also dedicate it to all those committed to healing and empowering children to overcome grievous calamity and win, and to all those who influence change.

And finally, here's a special dedication to the 4-A children whose courage and endurance amidst unimaginable pain and suffering have taught me the immense capacity of the human spirit. For our very survival on this planet, they are showing us the way.

CONTENTS

ACKNOWLEDGMENTS

I gratefully acknowledge and wholeheartedly thank my wife and three sons for their never-ending encouragement and support. A special thanks goes to David Harley for tirelessly researching many of the principle topics in the body of the manuscript. I am especially thankful to Gina Rumble, whose keyboard skills resulted in the timely submittal of every draft. Thank you to the staff at Charisma House and to Kathy Deering for their invaluable help in organizing my writings, and to my Integrative Medicine mentors and colleagues for all that they have taught me. And finally, to my ultimate and most consistent teachers—the 4-A patients and their parents—I am most thankful.

✛ ?! 㣺 ❉

THERE IS HOPE!

W hat has gone wrong? As even a casual reader or listener of the news knows, the statistics are alarming. Autism, ADHD, asthma, and allergies—all four of which happen to begin with the letter *A*—are on the rise, especially among children. In fact, it is not stretching the definition of the word *epidemic* to use that term for the way these disorders are sweeping the Western world. None of them are communicable in the classic understanding of the term, but all four sets of disorders, as you will see throughout this book, share common root causes that contribute to the development of current epidemic proportions. Autism, attention deficit disorder (with and without hyperactivity—ADD/ADHD), asthma, and allergies—these are the new childhood epidemics.

A tragedy of this magnitude would be overwhelming except for a salient fact: *these new epidemics can be defeated.* After twenty years of treating patients, I have found that beneath the surface there is an unmistakable, unshakable web of interrelationship among the 4-A disorders, and I have learned to recognize the patterns. Toxicity in the brain and body causes metabolic dysfunction, which cascades with other factors to produce one or more of these disorders. Often they overlap with each other in the same person. By uncovering and treating the common causes of these 4-A disorders, we can embark on a common (and hope-filled) path to recovery.

You are already aware of this epidemic, or you would not have picked up this book. Most likely you are a parent of a child (or more than one child) who carries a diagnosis of one of these disorders. You may be overwhelmed with your situation at home, while your search for help merely seems to bury you in information and saddle you with enormous medical bills.

I want to empower people like you—parents of 4-A children—with comprehensive and effective tools. With you, I want to advocate for the health of your kids. At the same time I want to increase your skills to recognize your own body's ongoing responses to disorder and stress so that you can make an ongoing and accurate assessment of how you're doing as a whole family.

HOLISTIC-INTEGRATIVE SELF-MEDICAL CARE

This book is a guide, not a cookbook. It will teach you principles as well as facts and point you in the right direction as you search out the best path. Recovering from any of the 4-A disorders is a journey, replete with side trips and even dead ends. But together with others you can make tangible progress toward the healthy, even contented, lifestyle you want for yourself and your loved ones.

What you as an individual do with this information is up to you. I want to teach you how to "self-practice" self-care in a holistic, integrative, and natural way. I want to introduce you to upstream medicine, in which we all play a role in searching out the causes of disease and eliminating them at the root.

The causes of this particular 4-A epidemic (and if I were not a pediatrician, I might add a fifth and more mature A to the list: Alzheimer's disease) are omnipresent in our man-made, inevitably toxic environment. The detrimental effects of our environment have been causing all sorts of damage and disorder that are initially imperceptible and can remain so for varying durations within a person's lifetime. In the case of many of our children the damage has manifested early on as the 4-A disorders, although some children escape.

All disease processes begin with changes in functional systems, imbalances that our bodies can bring back into balance up to a point. We cannot tell at first what damage to cells and tissues may have been initiated; for a time we remain unaware of tissue damage or dysfunction.

But after a point of saturation, months or even years down the road, a point that varies from one individual and family to another, an invisible threshold is crossed, beyond which perceptible symptoms of a disease begin to appear.

When I use the term "upstream medicine," I'm using it to communicate two ideas: (1) the way in which we can learn to trace symptoms of a disease back to common and basic metabolic roots, so that we can weed out toxicity and improve the health-promoting aspects of our environment, and (2) the way in which we can learn to anticipate damage or dysfunction long before actual disease symptoms begin to manifest, so as to keep our lifestyles as free as possible of disease-producing contaminants. An intermediate period exists wherein perceptible signs and symptoms of a potential disease are still "brewing," and during which, if appropriate measures are taken, the full definitive disease will never come into being.

MY UNIQUE QUALIFICATIONS

I am an established medical doctor with a pediatric specialty. As the parents of young patients have come to me for answers over the years, I became convinced that my medical toolbox was insufficient. I could help but only to a degree. Why should I spend my time and the hard-earned money of my patients' families simply trying to suppress symptoms of a disease, especially life-consuming ailments such as these 4-A disorders?

I needed to be able to do more. I needed to learn to bring together all that I had learned in medical school and in my pediatric practice along with as many other valid healing modalities as I could learn. I needed to become an *integrative* doctor, one who incorporates a holistic (mind, body, spirit) awareness along with a natural, nuts-and-bolts comprehension of basic biological principles. I needed to go back and relearn basic information about bodily systems (immune, digestive, nervous, etc.), in order to determine what it takes to establish and sustain the human body's natural ability to develop, grow, and thrive. Besides all of that, I needed to become aware of the bodily effects of our toxic environment so that I could make reliable recommendations to my patients.

In short I needed to learn to practice medicine in a way that actually eliminates the *causes* of illness.

This book reflects my journey, and I am very glad to be able to take you on board. I have written it to provide you with solid information, so that you can come to understand the causes and effects of your own child's health concerns—and so that you can move together in the direction of healing. You will find here a detailed summary of what I have learned and helpful applications of that information that you can adjust to suit your personal family situation.

A glance at the Contents page will serve as an introduction to the "menu" I have prepared for you. Some of the chapters may not apply to your situation, because you may be dealing with only one or two of the 4-A disorders in your family. But you will find that I have repeated key concepts throughout the book, so you will not miss them if you skip a chapter or two.

My desire is to put into your hands a transformational book, one that can transform your presuppositions and partial information so that, with me, we can create evidence-based solutions for some of society's most perplexing ailments. I want to bring you to the brink of discovery, where you can survey a variety of explanations and solutions and find the ones that align with your own physical, mental, and spiritual paradigms.

Each of my own patients and their families have gained greatly from what you are about to read. Now it's your turn to receive the same benefits!

SECTION I

HOW DID
THIS HAPPEN?

Chapter 1

❈ ?! ⚕ ❀

FOUR NEW CHILDHOOD EPIDEMICS

B illy was born ten days after his due date after a very long labor, and he had his umbilical cord wrapped around his neck twice. This did not seem to affect him negatively, though. At home he was a beautiful baby, always very active. All of his growth and developmental parameters were normal and on track. He was engaged with his family and communicative.

As an early toddler, however, he began to have temper tantrums and became very fearful of noises, which would make him cling to his mother for long periods of time. He gradually lost interest in his toddler play group. Billy continued to become more distant. Soon he would no longer respond to anyone calling his name, and eye contact slowly disappeared. By the time he was three, he had sustained numerous injuries while walking, running, or climbing, because he seemed to have no sense of danger.

All along his parents were reassured that their little boy's behavior was within a normal range for his age. And yet he could not tell them if he was thirsty or hungry, happy or sad, or why he was upset—it seemed that he could not convey any emotion. Also, he had had bowel problems since he was six months old, but his mom had been told that it's normal for children to have one bowel movement per week.

When Billy turned four, his preschool teacher suggested that his mother take him for a developmental evaluation conducted by a pediatrician. This caused her to begin to do some research on her own, and her studies soon revealed that a pattern of behavior similar to Billy's was typically seen in autistic children. Her fears mounted. Her Billy, who was once a healthy, happy little boy, now looked like a sad, helpless, clumsy boy who couldn't express himself verbally, who would get upset very easily, and who was losing friends faster than he could make them.

Refusing to accept that nothing could be done, Billy's mother located the website of the Autism Research Institute and found a holistic, integrative physician. He diagnosed Billy with autism spectrum disorder (ASD) and with severe food allergies and constipation, and he initiated biomedical treatment. Billy started a gluten-free, casein-free, and soy-free diet along with supplements that included probiotics, enzymes, and a whole-food concentrate (see Appendix D) to help turn around his "leaky gut syndrome."

After four months his parents could talk to Billy, and he would listen. Another practitioner was enlisted, and he diagnosed oral candidiasis ("thrush") and heavy metal toxicity. As Billy's digestive, immune, and nervous systems came into balance and his overall health improved, he gradually achieved developmental milestones in academics and social skills. Now he was able to make friends at school, to interact and play with them. He had good eye contact, and his speech was clear. Remarkably, he once again enjoyed life. He was back to being a happy boy who could tell his parents what he wanted.

As time went on, however, he became overly gregarious and extremely hyperactive. His mom remarked, "Well, it's just that he likes to do so many things. He's all over the place. He's a bundle of joy, but he can be very disruptive in a group." By then Billy was six and had entered kindergarten. He maintained good grades. The comments on his report cards were upsetting, however, comments such as, "Despite my best efforts I cannot persuade Billy to pay attention, and he remains a constant disruption in class." He was taken back to the doctor for a full evaluation. This time the diagnosis was ADHD (attention deficit disorder with hyperactivity).

What could have happened? Were the dietary and lifestyle measures that had brought so much healing no longer working? This prompted a systems review with laboratory studies, dietary history, and supplemental program analysis, along with a measurement of his toxic burden, which revealed that Billy and his family had lapsed back into a lifestyle marked by an inappropriate diet that was devoid of proper supplementation, along with a disregard for their exposure to toxins.

I am happy to report that once Billy's parents successfully reinstituted and maintained those lifestyle changes (nutrition, supplements, and a detox program), Billy no longer suffered from the effects of ADHD. As long as he stuck with the lifestyle improvements, he could be considered healed and healthy.

IS THIS A REAL EPIDEMIC?

We are living in the midst of a colossal, quadruple epidemic. This epidemic has developed insidiously over decades, and it has escalated rapidly during the past thirty years.

How is this possible? Isn't an epidemic defined as a specific disease that spreads rapidly in a definable geographic region? How can four seemingly distinct disorders (autism, ADHD, asthma, and allergies) share the same "epidemic" umbrella?

It's really not a stretch to call this a modern epidemic, even though the symptoms can vary greatly and even though the escalation seems to cover all of the developed nations of the world. This is because this diverse population of children (adults too, but these problems start young) are united in what underlies their many overlapping symptoms—and they face the same health-challenging environment.

We are involved in this epidemic with four faces simply because we are all exposed to the same cause. Toxicity permeates our eco-system. The human body responds to the threat in particular ways. When you add other factors of our modern lifestyles, you get a spec-trum or array of disorders that are interwoven with each other. The reason this epidemic came to light in children is because they are the most vulnerable.

Although we characterize what's happening as an epidemic, the children themselves must be evaluated and treated as individuals, because each person is affected in his very own specific way. We can see patterns and cause-and-effect, but many factors make each child's situation unique. Once we begin to understand where this epidemic came from, we next need to determine just where each individual fits. Only then can we pursue healing.

QUADRUPLE EPIDEMIC

Within the past forty years of medical history, we began to realize that not only were rates of autism, ADHD, asthma, and allergies growing into epidemic proportions, but they are also connected to each other at the root. Not only do they share overlapping symptoms, but they also often appear in the same individual.

My personal experience with patients and that of all the integrative physicians with whom I have worked is that we have not met one child who came to us with just one of the four conditions. The parents of a child with allergies would describe asthma attacks as well as their child's learning problems (prob-lems with concentration and attention span). Children would be diagnosed with autism and then with ADHD, and we would find that these hyperactive autistics also had severe

> ### DEFINITIONS
>
> - ASD: autism spectrum disorder
> - ADHD: attention deficit disorder with hyperactivity
> - Candidiasis (oral): Commonly known as "thrush," yeast overgrowth, or yeast infection, candidiasis indicates that the opportunistic *Candida albicans* fungus has caused white spots on the tongue and inside of the mouth.
> - Candidiasis (gut): Causing gut dysbiosis through the same process causing gut inflammation.

allergies and asthma. Our conventional medical categories consisted of separate diagnostic boxes. But these kids could not fit into just one of them.

> We have not met one child who came to us with
> just one of the four conditions.

How are these disorders related? What is their commonality? What element unites them all? The answer: the state of the digestive system. Every 4-A patient has an abnormal digestive system, which in turn impacts the immune and nervous systems, producing a familiar litany of symptoms.

"All diseases begin in the gut," declared Hippocrates twenty-four hundred years ago. He was describing our current epidemic.

CURRENT RATES OF 4-A DISORDERS

How many children have been hit by this epidemic? It is thirty million, when psychiatric conditions and the disorders in learning, behavior, speech and language, sensory integration, and motor skills are included. This certainly qualifies as an epidemic.

Is it an epidemic of genetic origin? While autism and the three other As have a clear genetic component, that cannot explain everything. These are not purely genetic diseases. Undoubtedly these patients were born with a genetic predisposition or susceptibility. Yet genetics alone does not cause epidemics, and it may not be as important as we thought it was. As Francis Collins, director of the National Institutes of Health and former head of the Human Genome Project, famously said, "Genetics loads the gun, and environment pulls the trigger."

Environmental changes occurring to a genetically predisposed child sound like a more plausible explanation to me. But what are the specific triggers?

I believe that environmental factors are of paramount importance. Autism has increased 6,000 percent in twenty years, ADHD more than 400 percent, asthma more than 300 percent, and allergies more than 400 percent in the same time period. Two disastrous environmental changes have caused all this to happen: overwhelming toxicity and nutrient depletion.

> "Genetics loads the gun, and environment pulls the trigger."

Maria Rodale, CEO of the family-named multimedia healthy-living company, writes in her book *Organic Manifesto:*

> Autism and attention-deficit/hyperactivity disorder (ADHD), diseases virtually unheard of a few decades ago, are now diagnosed regularly. Of every 100 children born today, one will be diagnosed with autism before the age of 8.* About 4.4 million children between the ages of 4 and 17 have been diagnosed with ADHD. Rates of asthma, diabetes, and childhood obesity are at all-time highs and scientists can't explain why the number of children with food allergies has increased 18 percent in the last decade.** Is it a coincidence that the prevalence of these problems has increased as we have increased the use of chemicals to grow our food?[1]

Toxic chemicals in our food chain are just one of the triggers. Let's take a look at each of the epidemic disorders in turn before we go on in the rest of the chapters to describe all of the possible triggers as well as specific and comprehensive strategies for dealing with them.

AUTISM

It would not be an exaggeration to say that autism affects everything in a child. Broadly defined, it is a severe developmental disorder characterized by significant disabilities in social interaction, communication, and behavior.

Autistic children range from those who appear to be normal to those who cannot speak at all or make eye contact and who engage in repeated and disturbing physical actions. In less severe cases children may be diagnosed with Asperger's syndrome or one of the other four recognized disorders at the "high-functioning" end of the autism spectrum. These children may have near-normal speech capabilities, but many autistic social and behavioral problems persist.

Autism affects about five boys to every one girl, and it is usually diagnosed at a young age. Autistic children have serious social impairments, and many lack an intuitive sense about other people, misreading social cues and not being able to learn from mistakes. This seriously inhibits normal growth and development. If they are verbal, some autistic children characteristically repeat others' words or reverse pronouns. They may have trouble engaging in imaginative play, a key aspect of normal development in non-autistic children.

Because autistic children can display such different symptoms, autism must be considered a "spectrum" disorder. Many people (and I am one of them) are convinced that ADHD carries the mildest form of the symptoms on the autism spectrum. Still milder would be "borderline ADHD" or various learning disabilities. Autism spectrum disorder is often referred to as ASD.

Children with autism, as well as those with ADHD, tend to suffer from asthma and allergies. Many also contend with other comorbid

DEFINITIONS

- Commonality: A shared set of attributes or features. In the context of this book, the word refers to an aggregate of environmental conditions and influences that have caused the epidemic of 4-A disorders.

- Allergy: An exaggerated response of the immune system to specific substances that normally pose no threat to the human body, involving the elevation of specific antibodies due to antigen stimulus.

- Asthma: A chronic inflammation of the bronchial tubes characterized by symptoms such as wheezing, coughing, chest tightness, and shortness of breath.

- Autism: A developmental disorder that encompasses speech development, social development, physical capabilities and tendencies, and cognitive development.

conditions, such as depression, anxiety, mood disorders, bipolar disorder, obsessive-compulsive disorder, sleep disorders, and more.

ATTENTION DEFICIT HYPERACTIVITY DISORDER

Like autism, attention deficit hyperactivity disorder (ADHD) affects more boys than girls. ADHD can be characterized by age-inappropriate impulsivity, inattention, and often hyperactivity.

ADHD is further subdivided into three types, as follows:

1. Predominantly hyperactive-impulsive ADHD. These children (more boys than girls) are in constant motion and find it hard to wait or listen. Instead, they act and talk impulsively.

2. Predominantly inattentive ADHD. More girls than boys have this type. They have difficulty staying focused and attentive, and they do not tend to "act out" or stir things up.

3. Combined hyperactive-impulsive and inattentive ADHD. Most children with ADHD have this type.

Inattention, hyperactivity, and impulsivity are the key behaviors of ADHD, although it can be difficult to draw the line at where normal levels of childish inattention and fidgety behaviors end and ADHD levels begin. These symptoms can lead to problems in academic, emotional, and social behaviors.

Sometimes other factors appear with ADHD and can make diagnosis confusing, such as depression, sleep deprivation, specific learning disabilities, physical tics, and overall behavioral issues. In fact, we find that most kids who have ADHD also have one or more significant psychiatric, physical, or behavioral problem, including bipolar disorder. Because ADHD has so many different faces, parents should always seek out professional help to sort out the reasons for their own child's behavior.

Although people with ADHD can become quite successful in life, the opposite can also prevail: school failures, discipline for unruly behavior, rocky relationships, and eventual substance abuse. Children with untreated ADHD can grow into adults who are depressed, anxious, minimally employed, and generally unhappy with their lives.

Throughout this book, when I refer to children with a kind of shorthand as "spectrum" children, I am referring to children whose symptoms put them somewhere on the autistic-to-ADHD continuum.

ASTHMA

The word *asthma* comes from a Greek word that means "panting." It is a chronic inflammation of the bronchial tubes characterized by symptoms such as wheezing, coughing, chest tightness, and shortness of breath. The inflammation is triggered environmentally by reactive substances or activities, including allergens, physical exercise, and cold air. The chronic inflammation causes swelling and therefore narrowing in a person's airways. Most treatments focus on reversing this swelling to relieve the labored breathing.

DEFINITIONS

- Autism spectrum disorders: Five disorders with distinctive symptoms of autism: (1) autistic disorder, (2) Asperger's syndrome, (3) childhood disintegrative disorder, (4) Rett's disorder, and (5) pervasive developmental disorder—not otherwise specified (PDD-NOS)

- Allergen: Environmental substances that are normally harmless but that provoke a range of symptoms in reactive individuals.

- Anaphylaxis: A severe and rapid allergic reaction involving many parts of the body, sometimes fatal.

- Bipolar disorder: A mental disease characterized by cycles of depression and mania.

When a person's asthmatic symptoms become worse than usual, we call it an asthmatic attack. Without treatment the person's bronchial tubes can close so that the person dies of suffocation.

Treatments include quick-acting medicines to give relief from asthma attacks and maintenance medicines to prevent symptoms over the long term.

Asthma ranks as the number one chronic illness in children today.

ALLERGIES

People with allergies have hypersensitive immune systems that react to outside substances in an exaggerated fashion. The word *allergy* indicates an altered reaction, deriving as it does from the Greek words *allos* (different, changed) and *ergos* (action).

Besides causing discomfort and illness, allergies can trigger asthma attacks and can contribute to the severity of many other disorders. A person's immune system is supposed to fight genuine microbial threats. In most allergic reactions, however, the immune system is responding in an exaggerated way to a false alarm.

Common substances to which people have an allergic response include pollen, dust mites, insect stings, pet dander, molds, as well as specific foods and ingredients in medicines. These normally harmless environmental substances are known as allergens when they provoke symptoms such as nasal congestion and sneezing, itching or swelling, rashes, digestive disturbances, or full-blown asthma. Most of the time allergy symptoms are annoying but not life threatening, although an intense allergic reaction known as anaphylaxis affects multiple internal systems and can result in death.

Allergies are very common in the population at large.

PUTTING THEM TOGETHER

In the next chapter we will explore how these four seemingly unrelated disorders, autism, ADHD, asthma, and allergies—each of which has mushroomed statistically in our lifetime and affect our children disproportionately—combine into one sweeping epidemic. I will offer encouragement to parents of 4-A children as I propose potential solutions. For the sake of our sons and daughters (who represent our future), let us not rest until we have brought this 4-A epidemic to its knees.

Chapter 2

✿ ?! ⚕ ❀

WHAT'S TO BLAME FOR THE 4-A EPIDEMIC?

The 4-A disorders—autism, ADHD, asthma, and allergies—seem to be distinct from each other at first glance, although the average person can usually identify similar breathing-related symptoms of asthma and allergies, as well as common behavior-related symptoms of autism and attention deficit disorder. However, the more deeply you probe into the details of each, the more you will see that all four of them are linked inescapably, and that therefore many of the solutions for these epidemics can be found by exploring the same underlying issues. We need to get to the root. While we cannot at this time repair genetic predispositions, we can certainly do something about the other factors that contribute to these disorders. As overwhelmed as caretakers and physicians can be by the chaotic demands of these 4-A disorders, our hands are *not* tied.

With the tireless efforts of many people, we have in fact begun to figure out the underlying causes of these epidemics. My goal is to not only point my finger directly at the underlying culprits but also to expose them to the light so that you can see them for yourself and learn to deal with them effectively. Regardless of your starting point, you can improve your family situation by what you will learn as you read this book.

Has your child been diagnosed with one or more of the 4-A syndromes? Which presenting symptoms are the most distressing and troublesome? Before you take off at a gallop for the nearest specialist, step back a moment and consider the bigger picture. We need to talk about how the human body ticks (or doesn't tick) and how vital bodily systems can get compromised. Then we might be able to point with more accuracy at the common culprits behind the 4-A epidemic.

FOR BETTER OR FOR WORSE: HUMAN METABOLISM

We all have it, if we're alive—metabolism. It defines you as a living being. In its most basic definition it simply means "energy in, energy out." Metabolism is the general term for the chemical and physical processes of a human body that convert and use food, water, air, light, and other nutrients.

You are talking about a particular aspect of a person's metabolism when you discuss breathing disorders; brain and nerve functions; digestion, circulation, body temperature, and body fitness issues; and even toddler potty-training. Most commonly we use the term *metabolism* to refer to the ability of a person's body to break down food and to transform it into energy. Precisely how each system functions is a complete subject by itself, but in general *metabolism* refers to the interrelated processes within a person's body that keep that person alive and kicking.

> ### DEFINITIONS
>
> - Metabolism: The chemical and physical processes of a human body that convert and use food, water, air, light, and other nutrients.
> - Metabolic dysfunction: A compromised biochemical process within the human body.
> - Immune system: A self-defense system designed to protect the human body from harmful invasion from the outside. The complete immune response involves many organs and types of tissue or cells, including the thymus; the spleen; the lymph nodes; lymphoid tissue found in special deposits throughout the body; lymphocytes (white blood cells), including T cells; and antibodies.

Well, alive and kicking to one degree or another. Metabolic issues determine how well the person's body functions overall. If anything compromises any of a person's energy-processing systems, it's as if the foundation of the house has crumbled just a little. The person might not notice it at first, because his general mental, physical, and emotional health seems to be just fine. But the next time that person faces a big storm (bacterial infection, accident, trauma, or the like), the foundation may not stand up to it as well as expected. Something may cave in a little. Something may crack. Further deterioration may ensue.

> We use the term *metabolism* to refer to the ability of a person's body to break down food and to transform it into energy.

So when we talk about any kind of metabolic dysfunction, we are talking about those places where the foundation has been weakened, where the biochemical processes within a human body have been compromised. As we determine what's going on with the biochemical processes, we can discover how to restore the processes to their ideal level of functioning.

YOUR BODY'S DEFENSE SYSTEM

One of your body's primary defense mechanisms is your immune system, which you might compare to the strong walls, windows, and doors of a secure building. Your immune system keeps intruders at bay so that your normal metabolic processes can maintain your health twenty-four hours a day. Our immune systems are amazingly complex and yet straightforward at the same time. We fail to appreciate them when they're working well, because they remain in the background, away from our attention.

If your immune system becomes compromised in any way, however, you know it. Many serious illnesses arise simply because your immune system has been weakened in some way. Some metabolic dysfunction has resulted in less energy for defense. Illness manages to get a foothold and sometimes takes over. Intruders breach the defenses, and now your body needs to put up a fight. We are all familiar with how this feels.

When we start looking at the 4-A disorders, however, we are not talking about an intruding illness breaching the insufficient defenses of a child's body. More often we are talking about an immune system that has gone into overdrive, thus introducing a cascade of physical, mental, and emotional difficulties. The child's immune system seems to be fighting itself.

Part of our difficulty in overcoming the 4-A disorders is that they seem so intractable. They always get worse before they get better—*if* they get better. As parents and medical professionals, we feel that we need to consider too many things at one time. Too often we fail to choose the right things to deal with first.

> We are not talking about an intruding illness breaching the insufficient defenses of a child's body. We are talking about an immune system that has gone into overdrive, thus introducing a cascade of physical, mental, and emotional difficulties.

It is my contention, along with other medical professionals, that we simply must look at the immune system as early as possible, along with the underlying metabolic dysfunctions, if we want to make any headway against any of the 4-A epidemics, allergies and asthma in particular.

T CELL TUTORIAL

When I say that allergies and asthma can result when the immune system goes into overdrive, I'm referring to the white blood cells known as T cells. The *T* is short for *thymus*. The thymus is a gland in the middle of your chest behind your sternum. The whole job of the thymus is to "train" and release T cells for the use of the immune system.

T cells are specialized. Some of them are cancer-killing T cells. Others help to activate the immune response in a time of medical crisis, and still others help suppress the immune response when it's over. Within those types of T cells we have what are known as helper T cells, and within the group of helper T cells (Th cells) we have Th-1 cells and Th-2 cells.

What do they do? At a glance (without adding layers of biological information), mature Th-1 cells attack pathogens directly, or they stimulate other immune cells to attack bacteria and viruses that threaten the living cells of the host. This Th-1 response is called cell-mediated immunity because it is performed by the cells themselves. Th-2 cells, however, do not attack pathogens directly. Instead they send messages to encourage other immune cells to produce antibodies, which in turn attack the pathogens—including allergens.

It's important for Th-1 and Th-2 cells to stay in balance in order to maximize the capabilities of the immune system. In many, many people they do not stay in balance. The most common imbalance favors the Th-2 cells, and it seems to come from stressors in a person's environment, including toxins. Yeast overgrowth can also shift the balance unfavorably. Toxic substances that can cause excessive activity of Th-2 cells include mercury, lead, and aluminum. These are "heavy metals" that do not belong inside the human body.

Overactive Th-2 cells put the body into too much of an attack mode. Allergies, weakened immune responses, and even autoimmunity can be the result. (Autoimmunity is a misdirected immune response in which the immune system attacks the body's own tissues as if they are pathogens.)

When the T cells are imbalanced in favor of the Th-2 cells, people cannot fight off common illnesses as well. Viral, bacterial, and fungal infections find it easier to attack the cells of their body. At the same time the overactive immune response results in allergy and autoimmunity.

Children who "get sick all the time" and who have obvious allergies almost certainly have Th-2 overactivity and Th-1 underactivity.

This means that their bodies are in "attack mode" when they do not need to be. Pollen, mold, and common foods such as wheat, milk, and nuts become like enemy invaders. These allergies result in chronic inflammation that can crop up in many predictable parts of the body, such as the skin or eyes. When the inflammation affects the bronchial tubes, we "upgrade" the diagnosis to asthma.

Do you see what I'm getting at here? If we can back up and figure out what skewed the Th-2 balance in the first place, we can make some headway against the allergies and asthma, not to mention autism and ADHD.

It can take a while to see results, but that doesn't mean it's not worth it. As you continue through the chapters of this book, you will see that I lay out a more complete program of detoxification, not to mention protection from toxins in the first place. I will also show you ways to help rebalance your child's immune system and keep it balanced.

Not all cases come from overactive Th-2 cells. Some children, especially autistic children, suffer from inflammation because of overactive Th-1 cells. Another type of T cell called regulatory T cells may help balance the Th-1 and Th-2 cells but not always. There is no magical fix, but the seriousness of your child's health crisis

---

DEFINITIONS

- Pathogen: A microorganism that causes a disease (i.e., a bacterium or a virus).

- Autoimmunity: A misdirected immune response in which the immune system attacks the body's own tissues instead of pathogens.

- T cells: White blood cells also known as lymphocytes that play an important role in the immune response of the human body. The *T* stands for *thymus*, the gland in which the cells reach maturity and from which they are released.

- Th-1 cells: Cells that can attack pathogens directly, or stimulate other immune cells to attack, in a response known as cell-mediated immunity because it is performed by the cells themselves.

- Th-2 cells: Cells that attack pathogens by sending messages to encourage other immune cells to produce antibodies, which in turn attack pathogens such as bacteria, viruses, and allergens. These cells do not enter cells that have been attacked by pathogens, as Th-1 cells do.

- Detoxification: Neutralization and elimination of external toxins that have gained entry into the body.

demands that you pay attention to what may be going on behind the troublesome symptoms of the 4-A maladies.

IT'S ALL INTERRELATED

Asthma is the clearest example of a Th-2-favoring imbalance. Autistic children and those who struggle with ADHD—who frequently also manifest allergic reactions if not also asthma—seem to be Th-2 skewed as well. So many of the autism/ADHD identifiers can be seen as the consequence of inflammation. These kids seem to have more colds and flu bugs than others their age. Their allergic reactions exacerbate their behavioral problems, contributing to distractibility, confusion, irritability, spaciness, cognitive sluggishness, and obsessive behavior.

It's not a happy situation. A 4-A kid is a discontented kid by and large. Hope is hard to come by. We need to try anything we can to help them.

FIVE ROOT CAUSES OF THE 4-A DISORDERS

Why has the incidence of the 4-A disorders burgeoned so greatly in the Western world in recent years, and why does it show no signs of letting up? Why are we seeing such an increase in these metabolic and immune system imbalances?

It's not just that we make more 4-A diagnoses than we used to. I believe the finger of blame can be pointed at four root causes, every one of which involves environmental changes. They can be listed as follows: (1) increase in toxins, (2) diminished ability to counteract toxins, (3) decrease in nutritional quality, and, somewhat controversially, (4) the administration of childhood vaccinations (too many, too toxic, too young). The spread of genetic propensity sets the stage, and the environment starts the action. Let's take a brief look at each one.

Increase in toxins

Sometimes it seems as though everything these days is polluted with substances that are toxic to life. Our food supply has been tainted with agrochemicals, artificially administered hormones, and antibiotics. Our overall air quality has decreased steadily, in spite of regulations and limits on industrial exhaust. The oceans stream with man-made runoff and waste products, and as you go up the food chain, the effect of mercury pollution intensifies. Drinking water, even sometimes the bottled water upon which many people rely, delivers unwanted contaminants. Maria Rodale explains how this happens:

> Currently, 60 percent of the fresh water in the United States is used for agricultural purposes.* And when it's used for chemical agriculture, which is by far the majority, all those chemicals leach through the soil and into the waterways and wells to poison our drinking water, our rivers and streams, our bays and oceans, and ultimately, all of us. Agricultural chemicals currently account for approximately two-thirds of all water pollution....
>
> Water is the ultimate recycled product. It rains, the plants drink the water, the soil cleans the water, people dig wells and drink the water, it rains again. The water we drink every day (even if it purports to come from Fiji or the Evian Mountains in France) has followed this cycle through the earth, humans and animals, and plants an infinite number of times. We rely on natural processes to clean the water. But neither nature nor our high-tech water filters can remove all the toxic chemicals from water. They build up and linger for a long, long time.[1]

One hates to become suspicious of everything, but sometimes it's appropriate. Toxins are everywhere.

Diminished ability to counteract toxins

A diminished ability to counteract toxins on a continual basis continues to be one of the five primary causes of the 4-A epidemics. The bodies of healthy adults can eliminate and counteract the negative effects of toxins from food additives, drugs, alcohol, microorganisms, metabolic waste products, and other contaminants. (This is never accomplished completely.) Children's smaller and immature bodies, however, cannot keep up with the deluge, especially when they have been compromised in any way. In my experience, 4-A children have noticeably impaired detoxification ability.

The information in chapter 11, "Healing Through Detoxification Therapy," can help turn this around for your child.

Decrease in nutritional quality

Without ingesting beneficial nutrients in sufficient quantity and balance, no one's body, child or adult, can maintain itself in a healthy state. I don't need to tell you that the diet of the average American child has deteriorated over the past few decades and that it has little to do with poverty or accessibility of nutritious foods and supplements. Quite simply, children whose appetites have been conditioned to junk food prefer junk food. Parents do too; it's the easiest, most appealing choice, given our harried lifestyles. After a while, our taste buds demand it.

Autistic children and those with ADHD are often very picky eaters, which adds to an inevitable decline in nutritional balance.

Even without a heavy diet of junk food, any child whose metabolic processes and immune system have been compromised will have "food issues," and only purposeful attention to nutritional quality can help.

Increase in vaccinations

Studies show a significant increase in the incidence of allergies and sensitivities in children that coincided with their vaccination program. The number of types of vaccinations that are now recommended for a child has doubled in number since the early 1990s, and although toxic mercury (in the form of the preservative thimerosal) has now been eliminated from most vaccinations, the damage was already done in children and young adults, and it's still used in a number of secondary vaccinations.

> Autistic children and those with ADHD are often very picky eaters, which adds to an inevitable decline in nutritional balance.

Vaccinations, especially when given at a young age, can make children more vulnerable to develop allergies by deregulating the immune system. As I mentioned earlier in this chapter, maintaining the balance of Th-1 and Th-2 cells is important. Vaccinations skew antibody-mediating Th-2 cells relative to Th-1 cells, thus disabling much of the cell-mediated immunity provided by the Th-1 cells. When a child actually contracts an infectious childhood disease (as opposed to being vaccinated against it), Th-1 cell activity results in a permanent immunity to that particular virus. But when children get vaccinated against the same virus, they never activate a strong Th-1 response. Instead their bodies activate too much allergic response (antibodies). Thus their bodies show a predominance of antibody-mediated immunity, which can lead to allergies. In one study kids who contracted measles were found to suffer 50 percent less from food and inhalant allergies than those who had been vaccinated against measles.

The increased number of vaccinations and resulting condensed vaccination schedule only added to the toxic burden in children's bodies. Here is a helpful summary by Dr. Kenneth Bock, whom I consider to be one of my medical mentors:

> The risks of the new vaccination programs were not brought to the attention of the public until...journalists and public health advocates...began to write about them....

When legions of parents began to complain that their children had become ill soon after their vaccinations, while still controversial, the government studied the situation and in 2001 began to gradually phase thimerosal out of the vaccinations. Even with this gradual removal, however, the damage was done. Now there are countless new cases of autism, with more emerging every day, and there are also millions of other children with very serious cases of the other 4-A disorders, which are also partly due to the unsafe vaccinations....

Despite all this, I am absolutely *not* anti-vaccination. I am simply in favor of *safer* vaccinations, administered properly, to healthy children, without thimerosal, over an extended time period....

The vaccinations...are by no means the only reason for the onset of the autism epidemic or the other 4-A epidemics. The widespread exposure to environmental toxins from food, water, and air are a huge part of our current problem. Genetics are also partly responsible, and so is inadequate intake of detoxifying nutrients. All of these factors, working together, created this problem.[2]

While the vaccination hypothesis remains controversial in some circles, I'm sticking with it because, in my view, vaccinations are guilty until proven innocent.

Role of genetic mutations

Researchers continue to discover how genetic mutations, whether inherited from parents or not, contribute to the incidence and degree of autism, ADHD, asthma, and allergies. However, genetic changes alone cannot account for autism or for the three other A disorders. As medical scientists are fond of saying, genetics only loads the rifle. The environment (physical as well as social) pulls the trigger.

ROUND-ROBIN BLAME

In addition to exploring the underlying causative commonalities between the four epidemics, we must also take time to point the finger from one to another, round-robin fashion.

> The vast majority of children on the autism or ADHD spectrums also have allergies. Many also have asthma.

Allergies, in particular, need to shoulder a great deal of the blame for the epidemics of asthma, autism, and ADHD. Pervasive life-disrupting allergies clearly have risen to epidemic proportions, sometimes proving to be fatal for children and adults alike. "How can chronic sniffles or a little skin rash be fatal?" you may ask. On that level they are not, although the reason we tend to discount allergies as a major problem is because they are increasingly common. Estimates are hard to come by, but figures that you may hear quoted are that food allergies have increased by about 700 percent in the past ten years and that about a quarter of all Americans (about 75 million people) suffer from some form of allergy.

Remember what I described earlier in this chapter about the damaged immune response. Naturally, allergies are not the only contributing factor to autism, ADHD, and asthma, but they certainly add to the pile of factors. In fact, I would go so far as to say that none of these three disorders can be managed or overcome unless allergies are addressed.

The fact is that the vast majority of children on the autism or ADHD spectrums also have allergies. Many also have asthma. Allergies are the most common cause of asthma. Ninety percent of all children who have asthma also have allergies.[3] A pregnant woman who suffers from asthma or allergies is much more likely to have an autistic child than a woman who does not.[4] In a nationwide study children with asthma scored much higher in ADHD behaviors, both cognitive and social.[5]

As the incidence of ADHD diagnoses has risen astronomically in the past couple of decades, so has the incidence of autism diagnoses. Can this be coincidental? I know it is not. Is it attributable merely to better diagnostic procedures or even to popular "fad" diagnostics? Certainly not. The children I see in my office are suffering from a complex mixture of painfully real maladies, and I can see the patterns.

The combined, round-robin blame for the 4-A disorders is not a chance happening; the situation is far too massive to be accidental.

A WORD ABOUT "REFRIGERATOR MOTHERS"

In 1943 Dr. Leo Kanner wrote the first clinical description of *autism* for eleven children who had been brought to him for treatment. He employed the little-used term that had been coined in 1911 by Swiss psychiatrist Eugen Bleuler. Throughout the 1950s and 1960s thousands like those eleven young patients were considered lost, abnormal creatures who would react to loving families with hostility and violence. They were not only hyperactive; they also screamed, rocked, and hit. They did not seek hugs; they withdrew when their parents tried to touch them. These children would stare for hours and look through people as if they were invisible.

The books of the time described autism as stemming from damage done by cold, unfeeling parents who permanently "injured" their children's minds. According to psychologist Bruno Bettelheim and likeminded child psychiatrists, it was the mothers, labeled "refrigerator mothers," who were the major culprits, subconsciously rejecting their children and oppressing them.[6] Other psychiatrists blamed "smother mothers" who refused to leave their children by themselves.

Finally, primarily because of Dr. Bernard Rimland's intensive fifty-year search of the scientific literature, it became clear that autism is a biological disorder, not an emotional illness caused by bad mothering. What a breakthrough!

Dr. Rimland made it definitive that a disorder such as autism stemmed from brain dysfunction, not from faulty parenting, and that, furthermore, the years that parents and their children had spent in psychotherapy had been wasted.[7] It is largely since Dr. Rimland founded the Autism Research Institute (ARI) in San Diego, California, in 1967 (directed by Stephen M. Edelson since Dr. Rimland's death in 2006) that the former "bad" mothers and fathers of the past have been able to get genuine help for their children. A group of researchers, scientists, and physicians came together in the late 1990s to found an organization called Defeat Autism Now! (DAN!), of which I am a member.

Along the same lines, in the early 1900s ADHD symptoms were considered to be evidence of general defects in moral control. In the mid-1900s, as doctors were beginning to try to understand them better, they thought that children with ADHD symptoms were minimally brain damaged. Experimentation with powerful drugs such as Benzedrine and Ritalin yielded mixed results, but at least we began to arrive at the conclusion that ADHD should not after all carry the onus of moral or mental defects.

Today parents of children with autism don't hear, "It's your fault." It took more than twenty years to overturn the old theories, in part because the theories themselves seriously delayed the discovery of the real causes of autism.

Increasingly, holistic integrative physicians and researchers are proving beyond a doubt that autism spectrum and ADHD children (as well as asthmatic and allergic children) suffer from toxic physical environments often coupled with genetic vulnerability. Now we can begin to move forward!

Chapter 3

WHY THE INTEGRATIVE APPROACH IS DIFFERENT—AND BETTER

My journey began with an early-morning arousal to the voice of the surgeon. This compassionate and skilled fellow physician had saved my life the previous day. "Well, it was cancer, Joe. We'll continue to get you through it."

I remember (too well) a tear-blurred vision of sunlight piercing through the majestic oaks and palms just outside my hospital window. One nurse-angel noticed and chimed in, "No time for those feelings, Dr. Joe. Remember, you have cared for my babies, and I need your help, still, to this day." There were others who needed me too—the love of my life, Carol Ann, and our three sons, Joe, Tom, and Marc.

My battle plan began to be formulated even before my discharge. The physician who would be overseeing my recovery happened to be one of the primary proponents of what he calls holistic medicine. He ended up teaching me a lot about the integration of the doctor-patient roles into a healing team and the importance of being open to all healing modalities. He also taught me the importance of having faith in myself, my treatment plan, and my spiritual beliefs because of the way this would increase the intrinsic healing abilities within my own body.

As it turned out, this illness has been one of the greatest forces in my life; it has strengthened and deepened me as a person. It was an inner process of growth more than an outer process of cure. I developed a pervading desire to heal myself from within, to change fear to faith, and to find meaning, direction, and love. As I participated in my own healing, I began to want to be able to introduce others to this new way of integrating physical healing with mental and spiritual healing—in the context of a community of like-minded and loving people.

CONVENTIONAL MEDICAL CARE

Conventional medical has developed very successful approaches for managing acute disease, along with a scientific process that is extremely efficacious. Yet it has failed to remain open toward many of the healing traditions around the world that have a variety of theories and practices that are successful for the management of illness, disease, and suffering.

Conventional medicine training involves diagnosis and treatment of diseases. The basic underlying causes of those diseases are not the major area of study. The idea that lifestyle could have something to do with an illness is not usually a part of the discussion, because this medical model is disease-centered and pharmaceutically based.

The list of advances in medicine made possible by science and technology goes on and on, but unfortunately in many instances, the human touch has been lost. Medicine has become high tech and low touch, and sometimes even the capacity for compassion has been lost. During appointments, the physician-patient encounter time has grown shorter and shorter. Physicians must spend so much time interacting with the latest laboratory reports and insurance requirements that they have little time to spend listening to and interacting with their patients. Physicians are under great stress; they report losing a sense of meaning and satisfaction in their work.

Medicine can be both high tech and high touch.

Medicine itself is in need of healing into its innate wholeness and power, direction and meaning and purpose. Integrative medicine is a major force that could do this. I firmly believe that medicine can be both high-tech and high-touch. A new paradigm is emerging. As a result of my own experiences as a patient, I now consider myself an integrative pediatrician, practicing integrative medicine as I see my young patients, so many of whom suffer from 4-A disorders.

Throughout my day I ask myself, "How effectively can we mobilize these children's nonphysical resources to enable them to live their best life, sick or well?"

INTEGRATIVE MEDICAL CARE

Models of integrative care have long fostered an understanding of the relationship between biological, psychological, social, and spiritual forces that lead to the disequilibrium we call illness. The balance of health and disease is a finely choreographed dance between our genes and the environment in which we live. The health of our bodies is part of a web of causation that is both microscopic and macroscopic; it links to the food we eat, the water we drink, the toxins in our environment, the emotions we feel, our relationships with friends and family, and our beliefs.

Integrative medical doctors call their methodology "systems medicine." Systems medicine is the study of the functional biologic systems of the body and the application of the idea that everything is related, that disorders such as autism, ADHD, asthma, and allergies never derive from a single process or dysfunction. The child's whole life from genetics to belief systems and how those influences are layered create a thing we call by a name such as "autism."

To ascertain causes of illness, we integrative doctors (along with the patient and, if the patient is a child, her parents) look at the five most likely origins of the illness: infection, allergens, toxins, stress (both physical and psychological), and poor diet. What do the symptoms tell us? What can account for them? How can we counter them? We assess the patient's real needs. Of these ingredients needed for optimal biological functioning, which ones do we need to give attention to first—food, supplemental nutrients, environment (air, water), rest, exercise, loving and health-promoting relationships?

Integrative medicine provides the instruments to shift from the suppression of disease and its symptoms to the facilitation and restoration of the innate healing systems of the human body. This good medicine of the future moves beyond the tools of pharmacology and surgery to the helpful modification of the infinite variables that create health or disease. This is new medicine. It allows us to modify gene expression (the way a person's genetic makeup plays out amidst the complex aspects of life) using therapeutic tools that include nutrition, exercise, mind/body medicine, nutraceuticals, and traditional healing systems. Integrative medicine focuses on the research and understanding of the process of health and healing and how to facilitate it.

Integrative medicine emphasizes relationships-centered care (doctor-patient). It addresses the art of medicine, which means it merges the human side of health care with the technical side of scientific evidence. An integrative physician develops an understanding of the patient's culture and beliefs to help facilitate the healing response, while focusing on the unique characteristics of the individual person. The doctor regards the patient as an active partner who is taking a personal responsibility for personal health.

> Integrative medicine focuses on the research and understanding of the process of health and healing and how to facilitate it.

Integrative medicine focuses on prevention of illness and maintenance of health with attention to lifestyle choices that affect nutrition, exercise, stress management, and emotional well-being. Integrative health care providers are encouraged to explore their own balance of health in order to better facilitate changes in their patients, requiring them to act as educators, role models, and mentors to their patients.

When possible, integrative medical practitioners choose natural less-invasive interventions before costly invasive ones. Using an evidence-based approach from multiple resources of information to integrate the best therapy for the patient, be it conventional or complementary, they search for and remove barriers that may be blocking the patient's body's innate healing response. They accept that health and healing are unique to the individual and may differ for two people with the same disease. They work collaboratively with the patient and a team of interdisciplinary providers to improve the delivery of care, maintaining that healing is always possible even when curing is not. They see compassion as always helpful even when curing cannot be achieved. Hippocrates, the founder of modern medicine, was an integrative physician. He stated that the job of the physician is "to cure sometimes, heal often, and support always." More and more Americans are seeking high-tech care from conventional practitioners, and they are also seeking high-touch care from complementary health-care providers, in essence creating their own integrative-care programs.

INTEGRATIVE MEDICAL PROVIDERS

- Emphasize relationship-centered care.
- Develop an understanding of the patient's culture and beliefs to help facilitate healing.
- Focus on the unique characteristics of the individual person and accept that health and healing are unique to the individual and may differ for two people with the same disease.
- Regard the patient as an active partner who takes personal responsibility for health.
- Focus on prevention and maintenance of health with attention to lifestyle choices, including nutrition, exercise, stress management, and emotional well-being.
- Use natural, less-invasive interventions when possible.
- Search for and remove barriers that may be blocking the body's innate healing response.
- Focus on the research and understanding of the process of health and healing and how to facilitate it.
- Maintain that healing is always possible even when curing is not.
- Agree that the job of the physician is "to cure sometimes, heal often, support always" (Hippocrates).

In short, integrative medicine aims to treat the whole person not just the disease. As you will see throughout this book, I see this as the *only* way to help 4-A kids regain any degree of healing and fullness of life.

INTEGRATIVE CARE FOR 4-A CHILDREN

In the past decade it has become easier to find physicians who practice integrative medicine. Increasingly, medical schools are including nontraditional therapies and integrative principles in their course offerings.

Still it can be a challenge to find a healthcare professional (whether or not the person has "MD" after his name) who understands how integrative principles can be applied to ASD children. Defeat Autism Now!, a group affiliated with the Autism Research Institute, used to maintain a list of recommended clinicians, but they found that they could not ensure the quality of every practitioner on the list. Consequently they now recommend that parents search for local clinicians via support groups in their own area.[1]

As a rule you will want to put some effort into finding a professional (or more than one) who can support all of the aspects of a healing program for your ASD child. Your own family doctor or pediatrician may be quite willing to collaborate with another who has made a specialty of understanding the complexities of children who have been diagnosed with autism, ADHD, asthma, and allergies.

DEFINITIONS

- Systems medicine: A study of the functional biologic systems of the body. The inevitable conclusion of systems medicine is that everything is related.

- Integrative medicine: Relationships-centered care (doctor-patient) in which the doctor seeks to understand not only the biological aspect of health but also the patient's culture, beliefs, and unique characteristics and in which the patient is regarded as an active partner in attaining and maintaining health through attention to lifestyle choices as well as medical interventions. As defined by the American College for the Advancement of Medicine: Integrative medicine combines conventional care with alternative medicine to improve patient care. Rather than practice one type of medicine, integrative physicians will often combine therapies and treatment approaches to ensure the best results for their patients.[2]

On the other hand your present doctor may resist some of the features of an integrative program, such as certain dietary changes or methods of detoxification.

Once you find the right physician, he or she will need to obtain a number of initial laboratory tests. The biochemistry of the human body allows us to monitor the function of its organ systems. Analyzing the quantity and quality of biochemicals gives us an accurate understanding of organ functionality—normal or abnormal, orderly or disorderly—and the insight we need to comprehend the signs and symptoms of ASD kids, to measure organ and tissue damage, and to monitor healing.

As part of getting to know a new patient, I usually start with a number of specific lab tests.

INITIAL LABORATORY TESTS

- Complete blood count
- Basic urinalysis
- Basic blood chemistry
- Liver function
- Kidney function
- Electrolytes (including CO_2 levels)
- Calcium levels
- Magnesium levels
- Blood sugar
- Lipids
- Cholesterol
- Triglycerides
- Thyroid function (including T3, T4, and TSH)
- Minerals
- Red blood cell minerals or whole blood minerals
- Plasma zinc
- Serum copper

- Urine organic acids
- Plasma organic acids
- Essential fatty acids
- Fat-soluble vitamins
- Reduced glutathione
- Lipid peroxides
- Plasma cysteine
- Plasma sulfate
- Comprehensive digestive stool analysis (or CDSA)

FURTHER TESTING

Food allergy and sensitivities are essential tests as well. Additional testing can include the following if problems have become chronic in nature. Immune testing panels evaluate the following:[3]

- IgA levels
- IgM levels
- IgG levels
- IgG subclass levels
- Lymphocyte subsets
- Natural killer cell activity
- Vaccine titers
- Viral titers
- Thyroid antibodies
- Anti-myelin basic protein (MBP) antibodies
- PANDAS profile[4]
- ASO titer[5]
- Anti-DNase B titer[6]

Each laboratory program is highly individualized and goals are mutually determined. All along, while scientific information guides treatment decisions, nutrition, spirituality, and other aspects of an integrative program will keep the healing effort holistic in nature, looking toward the healing of the whole child and the whole family.

Diet

Laboratory testing provides extremely important information about functional systems (i.e., immune, digestive, and nervous), helping us understand the real function or dysfunction leading to the symptoms that we are observing. Laboratory test data inform our interpretation and understanding of the child's symptoms and his likely reactions to various therapies, including dietary changes.

Here is where our little 4-A child will benefit the most from the team efforts of the integrative doctor working side by side with loving parents, who can make careful observations and execute the recommended changes.

> Our mission is to give every 4-A child his life
> back to the fullest extent possible.

For a 4-A child diet is all important, but each child's requirements are unique. You will find a range of information, sometimes conflicting, about diets for 4-A children. Food allergies, sensitivities, and intolerances are very common in these patients, and successful implementation of treatment programs is very often hampered by the "very picky eater" nature of ASD children. Some initial food-related testing must be done on every child while a treatment plan is being developed, and further testing along the way will be necessary to monitor outcomes (positive or negative). Diets should be implemented based upon your understanding of your child's individual metabolic problems. The actual diets themselves end up being experimental in nature, because only by using them can you determine which combination will most benefit your child at any given time.

HEALING FACTORS WORK SYNERGISTICALLY

The human body has been endowed by its Creator with the incredible ability to heal itself, but we have seen the formidable challenges our children face that threaten this healing power. Our mission is to give every 4-A child his life back to the fullest extent possible. Since every child is a unique individual, both the causes of his particular problems and the healing are uniquely individual and different for each child. Our hope is that the healing journey, through the development of an individualized healthy lifestyle, will lead each of our children into long, healthy lives. Four healing factors—nutrition, supplements, detoxification, and medications—need to be orchestrated in a synergistic program that is tailored for each 4-A child. Each healing factor has an effect on the others. They work synergistically, each amplifying the effects of the other. (This is truly a case of the sum being bigger than the parts.)

We must give these children what they need and take away what they do not need. The four factors, when combined conscientiously, are meant to do the following: (1) heal the digestive system, which will help to eliminate the major source of toxicity in the body, and (2) detoxify the immune and nervous systems. Another important intervention in the healing process is education, and as the child begins to detoxify with proper nutrition, he or she will be more capable of learning how to best live. As we will see, this applies to each one of us.

This is the natural, integrative approach to healing.

SECTION II

THE 4-A DISORDERS

Chapter 4

AUTISM

"My name's Jason. I don't wear Pull-Ups or have stomachaches or get scared a lot or get bullied. I don't bite myself or hit myself or throw myself down on the floor. I don't hurt inside or get upset because of it. I don't wake up at three o'clock in the morning and bang my head for two hours either. I have a bunch of friends, and I'm not worried about anything. I don't have autism, but my little brother does."

Who is Jason's brother? Georgie is a four-year-old with a diagnosis of pervasive developmental disorder and sensory integration dysfunction. His language skills are poor; he exhibits hyperlexia (repetitive speech) and severe echolalia (repetition of another person's words). He has other perseverative behaviors such as endlessly repetitive play patterns. He also has an obsession with trains. His severe mood swings and poor eye contact are only two of the reasons he does not interact with other children.

He suffers from chronic constipation, and it's impossible to miss his very strong stool and urine odors. Before each bowel movement he seems noticeably more autistic with increased perseverative behaviors and irritability. After bowel movements these specific behaviors improve considerably. Georgie has mild abdominal distension at all times. He has always suffered from repeated ear infections, and he had had nine courses of antibiotics in his first year of life.

Georgie and Jason's family background reveals multiple toxic exposures, especially before Georgie's birth. Their city is known for its polluted air and decrepit public water supply system. Around the time that Georgie was born, their father had been working in a gasoline station, their mother had worked in a photo-processing lab, and their family had been living above a restaurant during its renovation. Their mother had an unusually large number of amalgam fillings in her teeth.

Obviously the two brothers were developing quite differently. Although they belonged to the same parents, who were a decent, hardworking couple, something had gone especially wrong with Georgie.

In the suburbs of the same city, little Sammy was born bright and happy, the first son in a growing family. His mother breast-fed him and provided the best medical care available, including all the possible vaccinations he could possibly have. He talked, walked, loved, and played normally until immediately after his measles, mumps, and rubella (MMR) vaccination right before his second birthday. Suddenly he seemed to lose his language and became less interactive. No longer could he relate in normal ways with his parents and siblings, and he began to display classic signs of autism as well as symptoms of food allergies, including abdominal pain and foul-smelling stools. His parents were devastated. What could they do to help him? Was it already too late?

Jason, Georgie, and Sammy show us some of the facets of the autism family picture. It's a complicated one, made even more unpredictable by the way autism shows up differently in different situations.

As a pediatrician with a personal concern for individual children as well as their families, I am convinced that autism is a manifestation of an ecological problem and also, at its root, a gastrointestinal disease. I also believe that, as insidious and baffling as it is, it *can* be helped greatly as we apply ourselves to each child's specific set of difficulties.

A SPECTRUM OF SYMPTOMS

Autism is a spectrum, and every aspect of it should be thought of that way. Children with autism are affected behaviorally, cognitively, emotionally, and physically to varying degrees.[1]

ASD children have significant "systems" problems (digestive, immune, and nervous) that are metabolic in nature. These problems affect their physical and emotional health and their behavior. Even though their metabolic derangements are extremely complex, there is an inherent simplicity in the treatment. The integrative approach to biomedical therapies can take many trails that achieve the same result: clean up the gut and focus on what the child really needs.

For example, in autistic children, diarrhea alternates with constipation, with foul-smelling stools. Constipation is severe, usually resulting from voluntary withholding out of fear from painful movements, sometimes with only one bowel movement in seven days. These children are usually in a lot of pain from bloating gas. Being nonverbal, they'll express themselves with tantrums, refusing to eat, and "stimming" (short for "self-stimulation," repetitive body movements such as rocking, hand-flapping, or spinning that stimulate or distract the child from internal discomforts). Stool can become impacted and remain in the colon for months where opportunistic microflora can flourish. Liquid stool can leak through the impaction. Breaches of the gut wall occur and allow toxins to be absorbed into the bloodstream, causing symptoms in distant organ systems such as the nervous system.

You can't expect this extreme level of dysfunction to be fixed by a prescription medicine, a supplement or two, or a little dietary adjustment, especially since it goes hand in hand with substantial immune and nervous system disruption. We need "big guns," and lots of them, manned by people who have dedicated their professional lives to understanding and conquering autism from the roots up.

> This extreme level of dysfunction cannot be fixed by a prescription medicine, a supplement or two, or a little dietary adjustment, especially since it goes hand in hand with substantial immune and nervous system disruption.

Dr. Bernard Rimland, the first director of the Autism Research Institute, pioneered our current understanding of autism.[2] He felt the need to identify subtypes of autism in order to discover the underlying causes of recurrent symptoms and to determine the most effective treatments. Furthering Dr. Rimland's work, the current director of the ARI, Dr. Stephen Edelson, has described a subtype that has emerged over the past twenty years that he has termed "the medically fragile." During their first two years of life, these children suffer from digestive and immune-related illnesses.

My reaction to the following observation made by Dr. Edelson was one of the primary reasons for my writing this book. He said that these kids "respond well to nutrition-related, biomedical interventions, some of them improving to the point of recovery."[3] Who are the most important healers for these children, the ones in the trenches really "doctoring" them? Their parents! The burden that these moms and dads bear has made me very sensitive to their needs, and I want to provide them with ongoing encouragement, fortitude, and support as they develop the combined parenting, medical, and nutritional skills they need to bring their sons and daughters into the fullest possible measure of healing.

DEFINITIONS

- Hyperlexia: Repetitive speech.
- Echolalia: Repetition of another person's words.
- Stimming: Short for "self-stimulation," repetitive body movements such as rocking, hand-flapping, or spinning that stimulate or distract the child from internal discomforts.

The second major reason I wrote this book is to enable people to recognize their involvement in the autism epidemic and to initiate and participate in the healing process in their given circumstances.

Dr. Edelson developed a research project that included a visit to the homes of the families of ASD kids (hundreds of homes) to learn directly from the parents. He wanted to learn exactly what they did to help their children. It's important to make a point here. Dr. Edelson is a distinguished physician, director of the ARI, author, lecturer, and professor, and he wanted to learn from moms of autistic kids! He wanted to see firsthand how the children were feeling and responding. He talked and played with each child to determine how well they communicated, interacted socially, and used imaginative play.

> If we can further unravel the mysteries of this complex and devastating disorder, we can hope to make some headway against it.

With regard to their early history he found that 40 percent of the moms had experienced at least one complication during pregnancy, 30 percent had a birth complication, and they reported that the majority of the children appeared normal at birth and became "autistic" between one and two years of age. Seventy-five percent had a bad reaction to MMR, DPT, and hepatitis B vaccination (screaming and high fever). As infants and toddlers, two-thirds had eating problems (most commonly picky eaters), 90 percent had moderate to severe GI problems (diarrhea and constipation), and 80 percent suffered from illnesses associated with the immune system (i.e., chronic infections, asthma, and allergies). Dr. Edelson also discovered many communicative and behavioral problems among the children.[4]

His discoveries touched on a number of the causative factors of the autism epidemic. If we can further unravel the mysteries of this complex and devastating disorder, we can hope to make some headway against it.

I now want to take a look at each of these causative agents in turn, in an effort to help you understand where your own child's disabilities may have come from:

1. Good and bad gut flora

2. Immune system dysregulation

3. Mercury, other toxins, and detoxification dysfunction

4. Nutritional depletion

GUT FLORA, GOOD AND BAD

ASD children have severe digestive problems: colic, bloating, flatulence, diarrhea, constipation, and feeding difficulty. These problems start when they are weaned from the breast as babies in the second year of life. The children develop fussy eating habits, refusing many foods and limiting their diet to a few foods (usually starchy and sweet) such as cereal, chips, popcorn, bananas, bread, and other processed carbohydrates.

The gut (digestive system) is an open tube exposed to the pathogenic microorganisms and toxins of our environment. You would think it would be "gutted" by their assault, but the fact is that the wall of a healthy gut is covered entirely by beneficial bacteria packed so tightly that an impenetrable barrier is formed. The "good bacteria" protect the gut from outside threats. But if these beneficial bacteria are damaged, the gut wall cannot function protectively, and this can lead to a pathologic situation.

Here are the functions of the good bacteria in a healthy intestine:

1. They neutralize toxins.

2. They produce organic acids near the gut wall to reduce the activity of "bad" microbes; they keep the pH at 4 to 5.

3. They provide a physical barrier of protection.

4. They render pathogenic microorganisms harmless by producing various substances.

5. They engage the immune system to respond
   to invaders.

6. They chelate (remove, neutralize) heavy metals.

Without effective good bacterial function, the gut wall is vulnerable to invasion by opportunistic flora such as Candida albicans and toxins. Chronic inflammation can result, with injury to the digestive system.

Another function of the gut bacteria is to provide energy and nourishment for the cells lining the gut wall. If abnormal gut flora takes over, diseased gut wall cells result, which are incapable of digesting and absorbing nutrients. With normal, balanced gut flora in concert with well-nourished gut wall cells, proteins can be digested, carbohydrates fermented, and normal breakdown of lipids and fiber can occur.

Any damage to gut flora can result in reduced flow of nutrients through the gut wall into the bloodstream. Also inflammation from numerous causes can damage gut flora, which leads to "leaky gut," a condition in which the gut wall becomes pervious due to faulty barrier function. The result is that any food that is not digested completely or any toxin that gains access into the bloodstream can cause damage to the nervous system, immune system, or other bodily systems.

Essentially our intestinal tracts are a hidden ecosystem; we can call it a microbiome. This microbiome consists of over one hundred trillion microorganisms; our bodies consist of many trillion cells. We live in a symbiotic, macro/micro relationship (one ecosystem), where one party cannot live without the other.

In the microbiome of this corporeal ecosystem of ours, we find three types of microflora.

1. Essential, beneficial flora: These represent the largest member of microorganisms in a person's gut; they are critically important for exerting controls in a healthy gut (e.g., lactobacilli and bifidobacteria).

2. Opportunistic flora: These are present in limited numbers in a healthy gut that is dominated by beneficial flora, but if the beneficial flora is reduced in number or becomes dysfunctional, the opportunistic flora takes over, creating numerous health problems (e.g., clostridia). There are five hundred different kinds of opportunistic flora.

3. Transitional flora: These routinely enter the gut from the environment. They will either be disabled by the beneficial flora or prevail, becoming opportunistic flora.

Biofilm protocol

Many of the symptoms of autism, such as hyperactivity, aggression, and stimming are related to persistent gut dysbiosis. (Dysbiosis is the condition that results when the natural balance of bacterial flora in the GI tract is chronically disturbed, with a number of possible symptoms including diarrhea, nutritional deficits, and discomfort.) The biofilm protocol is a therapeutic approach to rid these children of this condition.

What is the biofilm? It is a collection of microbes, growing as a community, that form their own matrix in order to adhere together and better communicate with each other. In general biofilms can form on a variety of surfaces, but for our purposes we are referring to the biofilm that forms on the inner surface of the gut. There are two types of biofilm communities: (1) the symbiotic biofilm produced by the good bacteria that protect the gut lining, and (2) pathogenic biofilm, when the bad bacteria gain the upper hand.

In brief, bacteria out of balance result in dysbiosis. Once the bad microorganisms take over a GI tract, they are very difficult to eliminate. Efforts to restore balance include dietary changes, probiotics, and antifungal measures. Yet for many, many 4-A children, this is not enough. These children have GI issues that persist for months and years.

When those treatments do not work, it may be because the pathogenic microorganisms have been protected by the biofilm that was produced over time by the persistent dysbiosis. How can we tell if this is the case? Pathogenic biofilm indicators can be confirmed by a comprehensive digestive stool analysis, along with the typical symptoms seen in these children that result from the following problems: GI dysfunction, poor digestion, malabsorption, inflammation, and immune dysregulation. Treatment oriented toward eliminating the pathogenic biofilm can help restore normal gut flora—and subsequently improve symptoms associated with autism.

> Bacteria out of balance result in dysbiosis. Once the bad microorganisms take over a GI tract, they are very difficult to eliminate.

The biofilm protocol includes four steps: (1) using specific enzymes and chelating agents to break down the structure of the biofilm and to act as antifungal agents, (2) killing the unwelcome microbes, starting with natural antimicrobials then, if needed, pharmaceuticals, (3) cleaning the system with activated charcoal (charcoal absorbs toxins) to help prevent symptoms of bacterial die-off and to aid in toxin removal, and (4) rebuilding and nourishing the gut lining using prebiotics and probiotics.

Die-off reactions are almost inevitable, since you are essentially creating a highly toxic soup as you kill off the unwanted bacteria. This can manifest with symptoms of gas and loose stools, fevers, and negative behaviors. The pathogenic biofilm took time to form and will take time to be removed.

The bacterial population of the gut both produces and feeds on nutrients that enter the GI system in the form of food. So if dysbiosis is the prevailing condition, opportunistic flora will rob the host of vital nutrients instead of processing them and passing them on into

DEFINITIONS

- Microbiome: The totality of the microflora (whether beneficial, opportunistic, or transitional) in a person's gut.

- Pathogenic: The capability of causing disease.

- Pathologic, pathological: Diseased.

- Dysbiosis: The condition that results when the natural balance of bacterial flora in the GI tract is disturbed, with a number of possible symptoms including diarrhea, nutritional deficits, and discomfort.

- Inflammation: The immune system's protective response, elicited by injury, damage, or destruction of tissues. Inflammation serves to wall off the damaged tissue so that the injurious agent can be sequestered, diluted, and eliminated.

- Biofilm: A collection of microbes, growing as a community, that form their own matrix in order to adhere together and better communicate with each other. Biofilms can form on a variety of surfaces, but we are referring to the biofilm that forms on the inner surface of the gut. There are two types of biofilm communities: (1) the symbiotic biofilm produced by the good bacteria that protect the gut lining, and (2) pathogenic biofilm, when the bad bacteria gain the upper hand.

- Prebiotics: Foods that promote the growth of beneficial bacteria: legumes, peas, soy beans, garlic, onion, leeks, and chives.

- Probiotics: Foods and supplements that contain live "good bacteria" similar to those found in a healthy human gut.

the bloodstream in a normal, healthy manner. Even nutritional supplementation fails to set things right if the gut is inflamed and unable to process them; the pathogenic flora simply uses the supplements for food.

Nutritional deficiencies that result from damaged gut flora result in abnormal brain development and dysfunctional immune system in autistic kids. The typical deficiencies include vitamins A, C, D , B_1, B_2, B_6, and B_{12}; folic and pantothenic acids; essential fatty acids omega 3, 6, and 9; glutathione; magnesium; zinc; selenium; copper; and iron.

In order to even begin restoring what these kids have lost, we need to consider dismantling the pathogenic biofilm that has built up in their intestines over time.

THE DIGESTIVE AND IMMUNE SYSTEMS—HOW DO THEY CONNECT?

All living things must defend themselves in order to survive in an environment teaming with pathogenic microorganism and toxicity. The human body's defenses are organized into an immune system. An optimally functioning immune system is composed of cells and chemicals that recognize a foreign invader (known as an antigen), kill or neutralize it, metabolize the remains, and repair damage with minimal injury to us. This is done with increasing efficiency if the same invader attacks again. The first lines of defense are always physical barriers such as the healthy gut wall, which prevent further invasion.

If a newborn baby's gut wall is seeded with beneficial bacteria early on (the first weeks of life), this will lead to a very efficient maturation of the immune system. Newborns start out with very immature immune systems. If balanced gut flora is not in place by the first month, the baby may become immune-compromised.

The good bacteria lining the gut wall produce a substance called muramyl dipeptide, which activates the production of lymphocytes (immune cells) from the lymphoid tissues of the gut wall. Gut wall lymphocytes produce IgA (immunoglobulin A), which kills invading bacteria, funguses, viruses, and parasites, thus protecting the gut wall epithelium. However, unhealthy gut flora leads to a reduction in the number of gut wall cells producing IgA. The kids we are most concerned about, 4-A kids with abnormal gut wall flora, are deficient in IgA, which means they are liable to damage from the toxic environment around them.

Other immune cells known as macrophages and neutrophils are produced in the lymphoid tissues of the gut wall and also depend on normal gut flora to function efficiently. These cells swallow and destroy microorganisms and cellular debris in inflamed tissues. Also, healthy gut flora produces interferon and cytokines, which are regulators of the immune system. Conversely, unhealthy gut flora reduces the production of interferon and cytokines.

Another part of the protective barrier system to any invasion, working with IgA and immune system messengers such as interleukin-2 and interleukin-12, are the T cells and T helper cells (Th cells), which are found in all areas of the body that come into contact with the external environment. Again, with a healthy gut flora, the system works well. But if it is not supported by healthy flora, then Th-1 cell-mediated immunity fails, with toxins and microbes getting into the child's entire systems via the circulation.

The response to a Th-1 failure is activation of Th-2 immunity, which involves IgE. IgE is responsible for the allergic reactions seen in 4-A kids. Th-2 cells are also referred to as B cells (bone marrow origin). Th-1 cells are T cells (thymus origin).

In other words, as I alluded to in chapter 2, when environmental damage leads to the abnormal gut flora found in many 4-A kids, the response is Th-1 cell underactivity and subsequent Th-2 cell overactivity. This is also known as immune dysregulation, and it is partly responsible for the chronic inflammation and autoimmunity problems from which they suffer.

Thus, regardless of what aspect of the immune system we consider, we find that when the digestive system is compromised, the immune system is too.

Immune dysregulation

An improperly regulated immune system can be potentially harmful. Normally the Th-1 response is quick and efficient, especially against intracellular damage. Many of the typical symptoms of an infection or exposure to toxins, such as redness, pain, and swelling, represent the immune system at work, containing the problem. But if the Th-1 response fails and the Th-2 response predominates, antibodies can be formed against ordinary substances (which get identified as allergens) and even normal cells of the body, in an autoimmune response. What factors can lead to immune dysregulation? We know of four factors: antibiotics, drugs, diet, and diseases.

Antibiotics can weaken the immune system by exerting a toxic effect on the gut wall, altering its protein structure. The immune system attacks the altered protein, and autoimmunity results. If antibiotics are present in a mother's breast milk, they can prevent the growth of beneficial bacteria in the newborn baby's gut. At any point in time antibiotics can contribute to problems such as Candida overgrowth ("yeast infection").

Dysbiosis leads to immune dysregulation. Drugs such as acetaminophen and ibuprofen, steroids, and contraceptives can contribute to dysbiosis by disrupting the normal balance. Consumption of processed carbohydrates can also promote dysbiosis. Newborn babies get an optimal start in life with healthy gut flora if they are breast-fed. When they are weaned, however, poor diet choices can lead to gut imbalances.

Normal gut flora staves off the imbalances of disease. But the widespread use of antibiotics and a diet of sugars and processed carbohydrates have given opportunistic microbes such as Candida albicans a chance to flourish. This in turn can lead to what is termed "leaky gut syndrome" because the protective gut lining has been damaged. Partially digested foods get through into the bloodstream where the immune system identifies them as foreign and attacks them. Food allergies can begin here, although in most cases the body heals and beneficial bacteria regain the upper hand.

DEFINITIONS

- Antigen: (From "antibody generator") A cell or molecule that, when introduced into the body, triggers the production of an antibody by the immune system, which will then eliminate the alien and potentially damaging invader. These invaders can be molecules such as pollen or cells such as bacteria.

- IgA (immunoglobulin A): Produced by gut wall lymphocytes to kill invading bacteria, funguses, viruses, and parasites, thus protecting the gut wall epithelium. Unhealthy gut flora leads to a reduction in the number of gut wall cells producing IgA, which means less protection from damage from the toxic environment.

- Macrophages: Large white blood cells that help the body fight off infections by ingesting the disease-causing organism. Macrophages are "big eaters," named from the Greek from makros ("large") and phagein ("eat").

- Neutrophils: The type of white blood cells found in abundance in the bloodstream that serve as "first responders" when an inflammation occurs. Neutrophils are filled with enzymes that help them kill and digest harmful microorganisms. They predominate in pus, giving it its yellowish-white color.

- Interferon: A protein that boosts immune protection by interfering with the growth of viruses and other intracellular invaders.

- Cytokines: Regulatory proteins produced by the immune system to facilitate communication and interactions between cells.

- Interleukin: One of a group of cytokines (secreted proteins/signaling molecules) that help regulate cell-mediated immunity.

The gut and brain connection

Abnormal gut flora in 4-A kids produces toxins that have a strong ability to reduce secretion of stomach acid. The digestion of casein (from milk) and gluten (from grains), as in digestion of all other proteins, starts in the stomach. In 4-A kids with low stomach acidity, the digestive process goes wrong from the beginning, which sets up the formation of casomorphine and gluteomorphine, both of which are incompletely digested proteins that enter the circulation through a "leaky gut" wall created by damage from toxins secreted by abnormal gut flora. The immune system attacks these proteins in circulation, rendering them toxic. Their chemical structure resembles that of morphine and heroin. They cross the blood/brain barrier and affect areas of the brain by attaching to morphine receptors.

Thus, unless the child is on a gluten-free and casein-free diet (which you will read more about in chapter 9), gluteomorphine and casomorphine enter the circulation and act as neurotoxins to the child's brain.

Dr. Bernard Rimland stimulated thinking about autism as a biologic disorder for the first time in 1964 in his book *Infantile Autism*. He felt that the primary basis for autism is dysfunction of the brain stem. The Brainstem Hypothesis proposes that injury to the brain stem is related to toxins. One particular damaged and impaired area of the brainstem could account for many of the features of autism: the dorsal vagal complex (DVC).

The DVC may be vulnerable to toxins during the third week of embryonic development. The assumption is that autistic regression and loss of function could be due to poisoning neurotoxins entering the mother's circulatory system through her damaged gut wall and from there to her developing embryo.

Two brain stem structures that lack a blood/brain barrier (BBB) are the area postrema and the nucleus tractus solitarius, both part of the DVC. According to the hypothesis, this correlates with several features of autistic regression, namely:

1. The loss of vocalization

2. The loss of social function

3. Gastrointes-
   tinal dysfunction

The extremely high incidence of constipation, distension, abdominal pain, and diarrhea start at the same time as the behavioral losses (the loss of vocalization and social function). Toxins that gain entry into the nerve centers of the DVC suppress the generation of nerve impulses that establish normal muscle tone. With these signals suppressed, the muscles of the gut lack normal tone, so toxins can exert themselves in the DVC due to their ease of entry through the area postrema (AP) and nucleus tractus solitarius (NTS).

The nucleus tractus solitarius connects with areas of the brain that control social behavior. In addition, parasympathetic messages that originate in the DMV (dorsal motor nucleus of the vagus nerve) serve the muscles of phonation (the produc-

DEFINITIONS

- Blood/brain barrier: Separating the circulating blood from the actual nervous tissue of the brain, the barrier consists of the tightly conjoined endothelial cells that make up the wall of the capillaries, which restrict the passage of fluids (and therefore of toxins) from the blood into the brain itself. Two parts of the brain stem, the area postrema and the nucleus tractus solitarius, lack this protective barrier.

- Candida albicans: A yeastlike fungus that can infect the mouth, intestines, vagina, and surrounding skin. It normally maintains a small presence in the intestines, where it is not harmful. An overgrowth can lead to candidiasis.

- Gluteomorphine: A product of the digestion of gluten (from grains), a peptide that is known as an opioid because it shares a chemical structure based on morphine.

- Casomorphine: A product of the digestion of casein (from dairy products), a peptide that is known as an opioid because it shares a chemical structure based on morphine.

- Neurotoxin: A substance that blocks nerve signals.

tion of speech sounds) in the larynx and pharynx as well as the motor and sensory functioning of the gut. In other words toxic impairment of the DMV can explain the loss of vocalization and gut dysfunction in autistic children. In addition weakened muscular contraction in the gut leads to decreased bowel motility with resultant constipation and abdominal distension. By extension we can hypothesize that the same process leads to depressed activation of the eustachian tube muscles in the ear, leading to a high incidence of ear infections in autistic children.

So here we are, with toxins getting to a developing baby's brain stem, and from there affecting a multitude of seemingly unrelated aspects of growth. Incidentally, autism rates parallel the rates of increase of toxins in the environment. Also, localized autism rates correspond to proximity to landfills as well as local environmental cadmium and mercury levels.

MERCURY, OTHER TOXINS, AND DETOXIFICATION DYSFUNCTION

There have been suggestions that the vaccine for the rubeola (measles) virus might be a causative agent or factor in subgroups of autistic patients with developmental regression and GI symptoms. This is entirely plausible since several published studies have confirmed the presence of measles virus in the bowel tissues of children with autism, allergies, ADHD, and GI disorders. We must also note that, coincidentally, the MMR (measles/mumps/rubella) vaccine is administered at an age when most autism symptoms become evident (fifteen to twenty-four months). A live viral infection might just be the straw that breaks the camel's back. In a genetically predisposed, immune-compromised child with a dysfunctional digestive system caused by toxic exposures starting at conception, the development of autism is inevitable; if it does not manifest after the MMR is given, it would have later on with another toxic situation.

By the end of the 1990s there was an explosion in the incidences of autism. Parents blamed it on vaccinations since their children's health seemed to have deteriorated shortly after they had been vaccinated. The type of autism that increased most in incidence during this time is known as regressive autism. Children with regressive autism have no apparent symptoms at birth but begin to drastically deteriorate around eighteen months. As this autism epidemic was unfolding, so were the epidemics of ADHD, asthma, and allergies. I believe, along with many others, that these 4-A epidemics are also related, in part, to the increase in childhood vaccinations, with negative effects on the immune system. Two large groups of vaccination-free children, all of whom never developed autism, are the Pennsylvania Amish and another large group (thirty-five thousand) of children in the Chicago area. (Interestingly the incidence of ADHD, asthma, and allergies is also extremely low in these two groups.)

At the time thimerosal, which consists of mercury compounds, was used in the manufacturing process for vaccines and as a preservative; it reduced the chance of bacterial contamination of the vaccine. Evidence of thimerosal toxicity has been accumulating for years. Brain cells are especially sensitive to the negative effects of thimerosal. Dangerous effects of thimerosal on T-lymphocytes are well documented and include glutathione depletion and increased oxidative stress. These are immunosuppressive effects. Thimerosal inhibits an enzyme in the methylation cycle and depletes glutathione in brain cells. Although thimerosal has been eliminated as a preservative from most childhood vaccines, it must be noted that the way in which vaccines are administered (too many at one time) to children who are too young to receive them may still be a significant causative agent in the 4-A epidemic. For an extended vaccine schedule that I recommend, please see the book I coauthored with Don Colbert, MD, *Eat This and Live! for Kids*.

Mercury alone is not the cause of autism, which does not have a single cause, but I write about mercury because it is a good example of a toxin with a wide spectrum of negative biological effects, many of which are seen in autistic children. Mercury is ubiquitous in the environment. A major source of our exposure is emissions from coal-burning power plants. Once in the environment it stays there. Mercury enters water and accumulates in fish since they cannot excrete it. It is transferred up the food chain, and we absorb it when we eat seafood. Another source is dental amalgam fillings.

> Mercury alone is not the cause of autism, which does not have
> a single cause, but I write about mercury because it is a good
> example of a toxin with a wide spectrum of negative biological
> effects, many of which are seen in autistic children.

People with autism and people with mercury poisoning share the same symptoms. Dr. Stephanie Cave has classified the shared symptoms as follows:[5]

SYMPTOM	AUTISM	MERCURY POISONING
MOVEMENT	Clumsiness, slow physical	Clumsiness, impaired
DISORDERS	Development and difficulty swallowing	Development and difficulty chewing and swallowing
MOVEMENT CHARACTERISTICS	Arm flapping, repetitive movements, abnormal gait, and walking on the toes	Arm flapping, rocking, and walking on the toes
SENSORY PROBLEMS	Sound sensitivity, touch avoidance, and distractibility	Sound sensitivity, touch avoidance, and abnormal sensations in the mouth and limbs
SPEECH AND LANGUAGE	Delayed speech, tendency to be verbally inarticulate, and difficulty in being clearly understood	Loss of ability to speak, tendency to be verbally inarticulate, and difficulty in being clearly understood
COGNITIVE PATHOLOGIES	Inattentiveness, poor cognitive processing, inability to grasp abstraction, and poor concentration	Decreased intelligence, poor cognitive processing, and difficulty understanding words

SYMPTOM	AUTISM	MERCURY POISONING
PHYSICAL DISORDERS	Poor muscle strength, asthma, bowel disorders, allergies, dermatitis, and autoimmune disorders	Poor muscle strength, dermatitis and skin problems, bowel disorders, allergies, asthma, and autoimmune disorders

Toxins such as thimerosal disrupt the function of a key enzyme in the methylation process (a metabolic pathway that, among other things, produces molecules for detoxification and antioxidation). Furthermore, environmental toxins can suppress the production and reduce the availability of the body's most potent detoxifier and antioxidant, glutathione. By studying the abnormal methylation and detoxification pathways in ASD children, we can begin to understand their metabolic problems and susceptibilities.

On top of the toxicity of the environment and dangers of vaccinations, the bodies of ASD children have a decreased ability to detoxify themselves. Our very survival depends on our ability to detoxify. Detoxification begins in the liver and can be accomplished completely only with the participation of the detoxification systems of each and every cell. Detoxification refers to the neutralizing of external toxins that enter the body via normal metabolic processes. The process of oxidation forms free radicals through electron loss, and they are neutralized by antioxidants in the form of vitamins that donate their electrons, thus reversing the oxidation process. Glutathione is an antioxidant that often has a low activity level in 4-A children. When an imbalance in oxidation reduction occurs, oxidative stress results, leading to tissue damage. Consumption of antioxidant-rich fruits and vegetables can prevent oxidative stress-related tissue damage from occurring.

NUTRITIONAL DEPLETION

A final significant factor in the burgeoning 4-A epidemic is intimately interwoven with the others: nutritional depletion. Toxic chemicals have entered our food chain and water supply in unprecedented quantities giving rise to the chain of events (like an upward food chain) that result in 4-A pathologies.

The nutrient density of food plants is directly related to the soil; the organic matter, mineral composition, the soil microbes, and the chemicals used to grow plants all come into play. Not only has chemical agriculture devastated the nutrient content of our food, but storage procedures and food processing have also added to the depletion. Today's agriculture relies on herbicides, pesticides, and stimulant fertilizers to bring to market foods that are as much as 80 percent less nourishing than fifty years ago.

What we eat and how we eat are also relevant factors in health considerations. The American attitude toward eating has changed in our generation. Forty percent of American families eat dinner together less than two times a week. This differs greatly from a generation ago when 80 percent of families ate dinner together almost every night. A majority of Americans eat out five times a month. Twenty-eight percent frequently watch television while eating.[6] The environment in which we eat can affect our health and well-being.

DEFINITIONS

- Methylation: A metabolic pathway that is part of the normal detoxification system of the body in which molecules for detoxification and antioxidation are produced.

- Free radical: (Short for "oxygen-free radical") An unstable substance with an unpaired electron that causes random damage to nearby molecules of the body as it reacts with them in an effort to "steal" the missing electron.

- Antioxidant: A substance that converts free radicals and other reactive oxygen into more stable substances. The primary antioxidant is glutathione; other antioxidants include vitamins A, C, and E.

- Glutathione: An antioxidant, often with a low activity level in 4-A children.

- Oxidative stress: The overabundance of oxygen-free radicals in the body, which leads to cell and tissue damage.

Children in orphanages during World War II who received similar nutrients thrived differently depending on the emotional atmosphere they were in during their meals. Those who ate in a positive nurturing environment gained more weight.

These are just a handful of insights about the state of American nutrition today. See chapter 9 for much more about how nutrition can be improved to help our ASD children.

Oxalate control

Oxalate control is one specific aspect of nutrition that deserves extra attention because it is a new factor in autism therapy. Oxalic acid is the most acidic organic acid in body fluids. Oxalates are found in many foods, and autistic children appear to metabolize them inadequately; we can tell because we find increased levels of oxalates in their urine.

A brand-new diet is being extensively used to treat children with autism. This diet, low in oxalates, markedly reduces symptoms in these children. One mother described her autistic son as more focused and calm. He played better and walked better with a reduction in leg and feet pain. Prior to beginning the low oxalate diet, he could hardly walk.[7]

Oxalates in the urine are much higher in autistic children who do not have elevations of other organic acids associated with genetic diseases of oxalate metabolism, indicating that their oxalates are high for other reasons such as their diet or Candida overgrowth.

When calcium is taken in with foods that are high in oxalates, oxalic acid in the intestines combines with calcium to form insoluble calcium oxalate crystals that are eliminated in the stool. This form of oxalate cannot be absorbed into the body. When calcium is low in the diet, oxalic acid remains soluble in the liquid contents of the intestines, and it gets absorbed into the bloodstream. When blood levels of oxalic acid are high, blood filtered through the kidneys may combine with calcium to form crystals that may block urine flow and cause severe pain. Such crystals may also form in the brain, lungs, or joints.

Due to their physical structure, such sharp crystals may damage tissues and cause increased inflammation.

Oxalates may also function as chelating agents and may bond with toxic metals such as mercury and lead. Many parents who speak of their child's adverse vaccine reactions report that their child was on antibiotics at the time of vaccination. Yeast overgrowth associated with antibiotic usage might lead to increased oxalate production and increased combination with mercury, eventually causing deposits of mercury oxalate in the child's bones.

We frequently see autistic-ADHD children with oxalates from the diet or from yeast fungus in the gastrointestinal tract that bind calcium, magnesium, and zinc, leading to deficiencies. A low oxalate diet would be very therapeutic in such cases. I have described the low oxalate diet in more detail in chapter 9.

Autism is a very complex disorder, and the needs of autistic individuals vary greatly. After more than fifty years of research, traditional and contemporary approaches are enabling us to understand and successfully treat autistic children by taking into consideration the dysfunctions that are inherent to the disorder along with the particular toxic substances and depletions for which we must compensate. At long last, people—both the medical professionals and the hard-pressed parents of autistic children—are beginning to have hope. The symptoms of autism *are* treatable in more than a palliative way. Many interventions can make a significant difference.

Chapter 5

ADHD (ATTENTION DEFICIT HYPERACTIVITY DISORDER)

I first saw Bruce when he was six years old. He had been described by his preschool teachers as being a bright child but always impulsive, restless, fidgety, and unable to stay focused if he wasn't interested in something. He tested in the high normal intelligence range at school, and all physical health parameters were normal and/or appropriate for his age. At home, though, it would take one unfocused hour for Bruce to do ten minutes of homework. It was very difficult to parent him; he had to be told to do things many times because of the frequent fights he would start with his brother. He was in constant motion, and he couldn't sit still long enough to eat. He found it hard to get to sleep at night, and it was very difficult for him to get up in the morning. Diagnosis: Type 1 Classic ADHD.

Rachel's main problem was her inability to pay attention; for her, a few minutes of homework would take up to four hours to complete. After testing, the school psychologist said she was a slow learner who had only limited potential. With limited social skills, she kept to herself and appeared strange and eerie. She seemed to lack the desire to play with friends. She would forget to do what she was told, but she was not defiantly disobedient. In class Rachel found it extremely difficult to pay attention, even to her own name. She had to be called several times before she would answer, and she was always very disorganized. Her mom felt she just didn't have enough energy to get things done. Diagnosis: Type 2 Inattentive ADHD.

Sarah was a stubborn child who was known for throwing long temper tantrums if things didn't go the way she wanted them to go. She was argumentative and oppositional toward her parents. Because she was so easily distracted and/or would fixate on the work for extended periods of time, anxiously worrying about the quality of her performance and whether or not she would ever complete it, Sarah could not give her schoolwork enough attention to bring tasks to completion. She would lock into a negative experience and find it very hard to free herself from its damaging influence. Functioning socially was also a challenge. Diagnosis: Type 3 Overfocused ADHD.

Peter, age twelve, had a long history of quick-temper outbursts and rages that exacerbated his impulsiveness and aggressive behavior. His hyperactivity and short attention span caused numerous problems in school. Finally his antisocial behavior culminated in his attacking another boy in school, and he was expelled for the remainder of the school year. Peter's parents were incapable of controlling him at home. They tried one thing after another. Psychotherapy and all of the standard pharmaceutical therapies were ineffective. At last Peter began to show signs of improvement once the underactivity of his temporal lobe was treated with anticonvulsants. Diagnosis: Type 4 Temporal Lobe ADHD.

Seventeen-year-old Randy had always been a moody child with frequent bouts of irritability. His parents described him as never having expressed an interest in things that other kids enjoyed. His school performance had always been marginal due to his distractibility and short attention span, and now he was failing. As a result, he often spoke of being helpless and wanting to kill himself. He began smoking marijuana to feel more relaxed and less depressed, but this contributed to increased deep limbic activity in his brain and greater mood instability. Once he quit smoking and was put on mood-stabilizer therapy, he began to show signs of improvement. Diagnosis: Type 5 Limbic ADHD.

As many as twenty million people in the United States have ADHD.

Raul was nine years old. Very sensitive to noise and light, Raul had frequent mood changes, often expressed with anger and aggressiveness. During temper tantrums he could become very violent. He often appeared anxious and fearful of new situations, and when he felt that way, he would talk excessively and fast. These symptoms were superimposed on his core ADHD symptoms of impulsivity and a very shortened attention span. Antipsychotic medication along with methylphenidate caused vast improvements in Raul's behavior. Diagnosis: Type 6 "Ring of Fire" ADHD.[1]

IT'S EVERYWHERE

What's it like to live in an ADHD family? To experience trouble holding a small child because she is in constant motion? To chase a child through a store? To rescue a four-year-old darting across a busy parking lot? To experience angry outbursts with no provocation? To labor with a child for six hours to do fifteen minutes of homework? Many of you reading this know all too well what it's like, and all too often you have worn the label "bad parent" as a result.

As many as twenty million people in the United States have ADHD. It is the single most common learning and behavior problem in children. And as one of the most common problems in adults, it leads to job failures, relationship breakups, loneliness, and drug abuse.

Some ADHD facts: Many people with ADHD are not hyperactive. Instead they unjustly earn the labels of lazy and unmotivated, and they may be ignored because they don't bring negative attention to themselves. We are beginning to realize that females may have

ADHD in almost the same numbers as males, but they are diagnosed five times less often because their symptoms are different.

ADHD ranks with the most serious societal problems. Statistics are always being revised, but we can safely say that about 35 percent of kids with ADHD never finish high school. An estimated 52 percent of untreated teens and adults abuse drugs and alcohol. Something like 43 percent of untreated ADHD boys will be arrested for a felony by the time they turn sixteen. A number of studies show that 50 percent or more of prison inmates have ADHD.[2]

Seventy-five percent of ADHD patients of all ages have interpersonal problems. Untreated ADHD sufferers have a higher percentage of motor vehicle accidents and speeding tickets than others. Parents of ADHD children divorce three times more often than the general population. Although ADHD has a predisposing genetic component, poor parents or teachers can make the symptoms worse. In fact ADHD behaviors can make even skilled parents and teachers appear stressed and inept.

Although we used to think that people outgrew ADHD, we now know that many people never outgrow it, and they have symptoms that interfere with their whole lives. About half of the children diagnosed correctly with ADHD will have disabling symptoms into adulthood.

TYPES OF ADHD

1. Classic: core symptoms include hyperactivity, restlessness, impulsiveness, disorganization, trouble concentrating
2. Inattentive: not hyperactive, but with other core symptoms
3. Overfocused: core symptoms, plus trouble shifting attention and trouble getting locked into negative thought patterns
4. Temporal Lobe: core symptoms, plus severe behavioral problems
5. Limbic: core symptoms, plus depression, negatively, moodiness, and sadness
6. "Ring of Fire": core symptoms, plus disinhibition, too much brain activity all over, anger and aggression.

CAUSES OF ADHD

Functional brain imaging studies can actually show the areas of dysfunction in the brain of ADHD patients. Seeing where ADHD activity resides in the brain helps explain why it has such a negative impact on behavior. ADHD affects many areas of the brain, but primarily the prefrontal cortex, which is the brain's controller of concentration, attention span, judgment, organization, planning, and impulse control. Everything centers in the brain.

The causes and mechanisms of disease for ADHD are basically the same as those described for autism. Four causes stand out: (1) the toxification of the brain, which can occur in utero; (2) nutritional deficiencies; (3) autoimmune inflammation of the brain; and (4) inflammation of the brain from food allergies, sensitivities, and intolerances. I have elaborated on these causes throughout this book.

Toxification occurs because of environmental pollutants, including heavy metals such as mercury and lead. And because of chronic nutritional deficiencies, children's bodies cannot detoxify themselves in a normal fashion. Because of those same nutritional problems, they also suffer from impaired neurotransmitter function, and this is not helped by their almost-universal food allergies and sensitivities, which lead to brain inflammation. A large percentage of ADHD children are living with additional brain inflammation that comes from an autoimmune response to the streptococcal bacteria.

ADHD CORE SYMPTOMS

- Hyperactivity: Fidgety, nonstop verbal expression, difficulty with quiet activities.
- Short attention span for routine regular tasks such as homework, schoolwork, and chores: However, often a longer attention span for things that are new, novel, highly stimulating, interesting, or frightening. These things stimulate adrenaline production, which activates the brain functions that help with concentration and focus.
- Distractibility: Hypersensitivity to the environment, difficulty suppressing the sights and sounds of the environment, feeling bombarded by visual and audio stimuli. This comes from underactivity of the prefrontal cortex of the brain, which normally sends inhibitory signals to other parts of the brain to tell it to settle down.
- Disorganization: Especially poorly organized for space-time projects and long-term goals.
- Difficulty with follow-through: Unable to finish projects to the end (e.g., failing to turn in assigned schoolwork; putting off chores at home until the last minute or not doing them at all).
- Poor internal supervision: Again due to underactivity in the prefrontal cortex, which is the "chief executive" of the brain, involved with forethought, planning, impulse control, and decision making.

I am in full agreement with holistic, integrative medical professionals who believe that autism and ADHD are various manifestations of disorders that stem from many basic problems that are similar at the root. In short these patients suffer from complex metabolic disorders resulting from dysfunction of their digestive, immune, and nervous systems. The increased incidence of ADHD symptoms parallels the increase in the incidence of autism, asthma, and allergies, and this increase seems to track with the increased toxicity and nutritional deficiency of the Western world in the past twenty or thirty years. Modern biomedical interventions will undoubtedly change some of these numbers in the future.

> For all practical purposes, ADHD and autism should
> be considered part of the same spectrum.

Stimulants can be very effective medications for ADHD when properly prescribed, but toxic side effects are inevitable. It is to be hoped that the integrative approach to treatment will reduce the need for stimulants considerably. At the present time, however, the majority of ADHD patients rely on medications as their only means of treatment.

ADHD AND AUTISM LINKS

An increasing number of doctors, researchers, and care providers agree that ADHD and autism—with all of their variations—for all practical purposes should be considered part of the same spectrum. In my office I see a range of children whose symptoms are very similar, although to greatly differing degrees. In the same week I may see a child whose only problem is a learning disability, then someone I can only term "borderline ADHD," then an out-of-control teen with untreated ADHD, followed by another with Asperger's syndrome, and finally, a nonverbal child with full-blown autism.

When one compares traits between autistic children and those with ADHD, the similarities are striking. Both groups share the following, with the closest similarity occurring between children with severe ADHD symptoms and high-functioning autistics:

- With both ADHD and autism, most children have a poor memory, although some have a superb memory.
- Both can display notable mental gifts and skills.
- Both are perfectionists.
- Both can hyperfocus on a subject that is interesting.
- Both dislike change.
- Both have speech pathologies.
- Both have poor eye contact.
- Both have poor social skills and an inability to empathize with others.
- Both take unreasonable risks regarding physical danger.
- Both have involuntary tics and/or body movements.
- Both have poor motor skills (gross and fine), with poor handwriting, and an uncoordinated way of moving.
- Both have low emotional control, with angry outbursts.
- Both can range from hyperactivity to underactivity.

Many times it can be hard to tell any differences between these behaviors. Both ADHD and autistic kids have excess dopamine in their brains due to defective methylation (methylation breaks down dopamine). This provides strong support for the idea that ADHD is part of the autism spectrum. A fair number of autistic patients who have responded favorably to treatment behave and function in a very similar manner to those who have ADHD.

One simple reason that autism and ADHD tend to be viewed as distinct from each other is because of the psychiatric diagnostic system, by which a person is limited to one primary diagnosis of her prevailing (or most severe) disorder. So if a child has major symptoms for autism along with comparatively minor symptoms of ADHD, the basic diagnosis will be autism. Why should this matter? It shouldn't if treatment decision makers recognize the underlying link between ADHD and autism and explore many options that might work for either/both. But treatment options tend to be limited to the ones that are favored for one or the other disorder.

In addition both disorders seem to be linked by the same comorbid disorders. Not all children have all of these additional disorders, of course. It's just that many, many children and adults who have been diagnosed with ADHD or autism also have one of the following psychological or neurological problems: depression, anxiety disorders, mood disorders, bipolar disorder, obsessive-compulsive disorder (OCD), oppositional defiant disorder (ODD), learning and/or speech disabilities, sleep disorders such as insomnia, and communication disorders such as the inability to pronounce certain sounds or stuttering.

> ## DEFINITIONS
>
> - ADHD (attention deficit hyperactivity disorder): A neurobehavioral disorder marked by varying degrees and types of impulsivity, inattentiveness, and/or hyperactivity.
> - Methylphenidate: The most common class of ADHD drugs (includes Ritalin). The effects of methylphenidates are similar to those of amphetamines, only milder, and they can help calm children with ADHD.
> - Dopamine: A neurotransmitter that contributes to positive mood, energy level, and physical grace, often found in abnormal levels in ASD children.

TREATING YOUR CHILD'S ADHD

You will find more specifics about treating your child's ADHD in the third section of this book, "Healing Therapies for the 4-A Disorders."

In general you should know that the best treatment is a combination of medication, counseling, lifestyle changes (especially dietary changes), and behavior modification. Medication is usually indicated, at least for a period of time, in order to enable the child's behavior to improve enough to allow success in other efforts. Still, medication is not a cure for ADHD, and guidelines for their usage vary.

Increasingly, school staffs and medical professionals are recognizing the ADHD epidemic as a valid problem and are educating themselves about how to best enable the ADHD children in their care to thrive. Many of them have become skilled in particular therapeutic approaches and may well be of significant assistance in your own situation.

You might seek out a support group, either locally or online, to help you maintain your perspective and energy as you make friends with other parents of ADHD children.

Above all you must learn to value the idea of your active partnership with your medical professionals, teachers and aides, and regular caregivers. You, as the parent, will be the best one to assess the ongoing situation, to make decisions, and to carry them through. As you target specific, situation-appropriate goals for finite stretches of time, you will be the one making the meals, dispensing the medication, and supporting behavior therapy and other therapies. You will be the best one to limit distractions in your child's daily life, to make sure that the daily schedule is as predictable as possible, to set and maintain healthy parameters of behavior with appropriate discipline, and to spot the smallest praiseworthy moments. You will be the one to follow up on a regular basis with the pediatrician or other clinical professional. You will be the one to love your child unconditionally and to afford for him or her every possible chance to live a long and happy life.

Chapter 6

THE ASTHMA EPIDEMIC

Seven-year-old John was brought to my office because of a problem that he had never experienced before. His mother explained that he had come down with a simple cold, but now he was having difficulty breathing.

His skin was pale, and he appeared frightened as he labored to breathe, panting as he tried to get air into his lungs. He seemed to have even more difficulty getting it out. The skin retracting between his ribs and above his clavicles was moist with sweat. He had a "tight," muffled cough that made him wince with pain. He looked exhausted as he sat with slumped shoulders on my exam table. When I listened to his lungs with my stethoscope, I could hear whistles and high-pitched noises—better known as wheezing—bilaterally (in both lung fields).

I explained to John's mom that her son was having an acute episode of bronchospasm, a tightening of the muscles lining the walls of his bronchial (breathing) tubes, and that this severely narrowed the space for air to pass. He also had inflammatory swelling of the mucous membrane that lines the inside of the tubes. Further I explained that if this attack recurred and if these attacks responded positively to bronchodilators and anti-inflammatory medicine, then I would likely make a diagnosis of asthma.

Three months later John returned with the same symptoms after playing basketball all day. I explained that exercise-induced bronchospasm provokes the same reaction as when he had the cold virus and that he should be treated in a similar fashion as before. I also explained that if this happens repeatedly, John's lungs will sustain damage.

A TRUE EPIDEMIC

Asthma is on the rise. Approximately 34.1 million men, women, and children in the United States have been diagnosed with chronic asthma, and if you add the number of asthma sufferers from around the globe, the number rises to 300 million.[1] The prevalence of asthma increased by 75 percent between 1980 and 1994.[2] In 2007 alone 185 children and 3,262 adults died from asthma.[3]

As Dr. Kenneth Bock observes in *Healing the New Childhood Epidemics*:

> Fatalities from asthma are now twice as common as they were in 1980, despite advances in hospital crisis care. The main reason for this is simply that during this period the incidence of asthma tripled. In addition, more people have very serious cases of asthma.
>
> Without question, we are in the depths of history's worst epidemic of asthma.[4]

Let's take a look at some further statistics that pertain specifically to children:

- Nine million Americans eighteen or younger have asthma.

- In high-incidence zones, such as the Bronx or Central Harlem in New York City, up to 25 percent of all children now have asthma.

- In very large regions of high incidence—including New Jersey, New England, and New York—12 percent to 15 percent of all children have asthma.

- Children who take antibiotics before age four have 400 percent more asthma than others.

- Approximately 40 percent of asthmatic adults have asthmatic children.

- Asthma causes 14 million missed school days each year.[5]

Asthma is the number one chronic respiratory disease in the United States. It is a disease of the lungs, and the term *asthma* comes from the Greek word for "panting." People with asthma pant because they find it so difficult to breathe. When they are experiencing an attack, the tubes inside their lungs that deliver air (the bronchi) become inflamed, and the muscles of the bronchial walls tighten or spasm. Extra mucus gets produced, which further congests and narrows the airways. These obstructive changes leave very little room for air to get through.

The severity of the attack can vary from slight wheezing to life threatening. John's attack was somewhere in between. In more severe attacks people often panic because of the feeling of strangulation. Deprived of oxygen, they can become dizzy and confused, and they can vomit. After becoming pale their extremities and lips can begin to turn blue. Without medical intervention a prolonged attack exhausts the person, often to the point of losing their battle with suffocation.

Asthma is the number one chronic respiratory disease in the United States.

Is this the worst asthma epidemic in history? Undoubtedly it is! With the highest incidence occurring within the past thirty years, nine million of whom are pediatric patients, asthma is the leading cause of hospitalizations for youth, as well as school absenteeism.

This high incidence coincides with the equally steep rise in the incidence of autism, ADHD, and allergies during the same time period. Is this a mere coincidence? As you know by now from having read the earlier chapters of this book, these conditions are not isolated from one another at all. In fact, they seem to share the common traits of genetic predisposition, nutritional deficiencies, and reactions to toxic environmental exposure.

DEFINITIONS

- Bronchospasm: A term descriptive of asthma, namely a constriction of the muscles of the bronchial walls that causes labored breathing, wheezing, and other symptoms. Children and adults with asthma can develop bronchospasm symptoms when they get exposed to any one of a number of triggers (e.g., exercise, especially in cool weather outdoors; a virus; an allergen; or an irritant).

- Bronchodilator: A drug that, when inhaled for the relief of an asthma attack, relaxes the constricted bronchial muscles and thereby causes the bronchial tubes to widen. Short-acting bronchodilators help during asthma attacks, and long-acting types need to be taken daily, often with a steroid.

DYSFUNCTIONAL IMMUNE SYSTEMS AND INFLAMMATION

The inflammation of the airways in asthma is actually a dysfunction of the immune system. Basically, overactivity of the immune system leads to asthma. In particular it is the T cells' and lymphocytes' overactivity. A dysfunctional immune system gives rise to allergies, which are the major cause of asthma. Almost all children with asthma also have allergies. Autistic children have ADHD traits, allergies, and, frequently, asthma. More than 75 percent of the time asthmatics also suffer from gastroesophageal reflux, which is a common symptom of food allergies.

In chapter 2 I described at some length the way the immune system works. You might want to glance back at the information about T cells in order to review the reasons for the skewing of the Th-2 antibody production and the resulting impaired immune response. An overactive Th-2 immune response means that a person's immune system ends up considering ordinary substances allergens, such as common foods and pollens. Inflammation (nose, eye, skin, etc.) is the symptomatic result of the allergic response, and quite often that inflammation occurs in the bronchial tubes. What's the result? All too often asthma. Allergies are known to be the single most common trigger for asthma.

If you are the parent of a child on the autism spectrum and/or with ADHD, you already know from firsthand experience that your child tends to catch every "bug" that comes along. You also know how hard it can be to sort out some of your child's neurobehavioral traits (such as irritability, mental sluggishness, and spaciness). How much can you blame on allergies? How can you separate the allergies and asthma from the ADHD or autism symptoms?

I do not have an easy answer for you; I wish I did. The four disorders present themselves as a tangled mess, with asthma too often right in the middle.

TREATMENTS FOR ASTHMA

As with the other three of the epidemic disorders, asthma can be greatly helped, if not alleviated, by diligent attention to the root causes of the immune dysfunction and the body's reaction to toxic substances. However, in the case of asthma, the first line of defense *must* be medicines. Your child's very survival may depend on it.

Asthma drugs—principally anti-inflammatories and bronchodilators—do not cure the disease, but they keep the symptoms under control as you determine what else to do for your child. You can read much more about how these medicines are administered in chapter 12, under the section entitled "Medications for Asthma."

> In the case of asthma, the first line of defense *must* be medicines. Your child's very survival may depend on it.

As I note in that chapter, the best treatment aims to prevent asthma attacks if at all possible, and medicating a child as early as possible when an attack occurs, before the bronchial spasms become more severe. You will want to pay particular attention to allergies and other sources of irritation and inflammation. Beyond the obvious airborne potential allergens and irritants you will want to try to determine foods and other sources of trouble. The elimination diets in chapter 9 may prove to be helpful to you.

Alternative therapies, which you may or may not decide to have your child undertake, include acupuncture, biofeedback, chiropractic adjustments, hypnosis, laser therapy to shrink swollen tissues, and various relaxation techniques for reducing stress and anxiety (because stress and anxiety can contribute to asthma symptoms). I have expounded upon this list of alternative therapies in Appendix C, "Additional Therapies for Asthma and Allergies."

SELECTED ALTERNATIVE THERAPIES FOR ASTHMA[6]

- Acupuncture: A technique that involves inserting needles into key points of the body. Evidence suggests that acupuncture may signal the brain to release endorphins. These are hormones made by the body. When released, endorphins can help reduce pain and create a sense of well-being. People with asthma or allergies may experience more relaxed or calmer breathing.

- Biofeedback: A technique that helps people control involuntary physical responses. Results are mixed, with children and teenagers showing the greatest benefit.

- Chiropractic spinal manipulation: A technique that emphasizes manipulation of the spine in order to help the body heal itself. There is no evidence that this treatment impairs the underlying disease or pulmonary function.

- Hypnosis: An artificially induced dream state that leaves the person open to suggestion. Hypnosis might give people with asthma or allergies more self-discipline to follow good health practices.

- Laser treatment: A technique that uses high-intensity light to shrink swollen tissue or to unblock sinuses. Laser therapy may provide temporary relief, but it may also cause scarring or other long-term physical problems.

- Massage, relaxation techniques, art/music therapy, yoga: Stress and anxiety may cause your airways to constrict more if you have asthma or allergies. Various techniques can help you relax, reduce anxiety, or control your breathing. The results may provide some benefit in helping you cope with asthma or allergy symptoms.

GETTING ON TOP OF ASTHMA

Asthma is not usually a solo disorder. In fact, we have seen its rise parallel the rise in autism, ADHD, and allergies precisely because it often appears in the same immune-compromised individuals.

Although it does not appear out of nowhere as a primary diagnosis, asthma can be a serious enough ailment to command more than its share of parental and professional resources. If your child suffers from asthma as well as from significant allergies and perhaps ADHD or autism, you have your hands full. You welcome anything that can bring a sense of order to the chaos and complexity of your family life, and you may have almost despaired of being able to conquer the situation.

Speaking to you as an empathetic physician, I must tell you that the *only* way you will be able to follow a treatment program that will eliminate false leads and take you as far as possible down the road to healing will be to immerse yourself in the information in this book and similar resources.

You have been living the 4-A epidemic in your own home. Now it's time to start living the healing of it.

Chapter 7

ALLERGIES—THE UNIVERSAL THREAT

Patrick is sixteen years old, and he has a history of allergies with frequent bouts of coughing. One breezy day an allergic reaction localized in his airways. By himself he stumbled into my office, gasping for air. He whispered that he felt as if he was being strangled, and he complained of dizziness. He looked disoriented. Suddenly he vomited, and he began to panic as his skin began to turn bluish, and he became drenched with sweat. After a subcutaneous injection of epinephrine, I placed an endotracheal tube into his trachea and applied 100 percent oxygen as my nurse opened a vein for intravenous bronchodilators. Finally Patrick began to rest comfortably. Diagnosis: severe allergic asthma.

William, age four, has autism spectrum disorder (ASD), and five months of specific therapies had brought much progress. His mother described in detail how well he had progressed in his language skills, sensory issues, motor skills, digestive function, and learning-processing capabilities. His program for healing included nutritional supplementation and detoxification protocols that had been implemented in the most compliant manner, along with applied behavioral analysis and other specific therapies. William was very successfully moving into the mainstream—until it all came crashing down over the course of one weekend. His mother had brought him in because William had reverted back to his ASD symptoms as if no therapy had ever been started. By means of simple queries I found out that William had eaten foods that he was allergic to during the weekend. That's all; nothing else had changed. Diagnosis: ASD and food allergy.

Practically all 4-A children have serious allergies, in my estimation. Allergies are among the most powerful and destructive of all the interwoven forces that compose these childhood epidemics, and they contribute immeasurably to the scourges of autism, ADHD, and asthma.

Of course allergies constitute an epidemic in their own right. Food allergies have increased several hundredfold in the past ten years, and fatal allergic reactions seem to be far more common than ever before. Easily a quarter (probably much more) of the American population has allergies, including the vast majority of all children with autism, ADHD, and asthma.

What are people allergic to? Just about everything. They are allergic to inhalants such as plant pollen, animal dander, mold spores, vehicle exhaust, and the fumes of chemical products such as paint and cleaning solutions. They react to insect stings, antibiotics, and many drugs. Some people have allergic reactions to touching certain plants, wearing jewelry made of certain substances, and using makeup or other beauty products. Emerging as bigger than we thought are allergies to foods, especially to peanuts, shellfish, eggs, and milk.

What we're not allergic to, we often have sensitivities to or intolerances for. The problem will continue to increase. We need to find out how to deal with it where it touches our own lives.

TYPES OF ALLERGENS

- Inhalants: plant pollen, animal dander, mold spores, vehicle exhaust, and chemical products (paint, cleaning solutions)
- Ingestants (food): milk, egg, peanuts, wheat, fish
- Medications: antibiotics, nonsteroid anti-inflammatory
- Contactants: plants, jewelry, beauty products
- Injectants: insect stings

COMMON ALLERGY AND SENSITIVITY SYMPTOMS

Because allergies are so common, many people do not consider allergies dangerous, and they associate allergies with the mildest of symptoms, such as a runny nose. Yet any symptom can be caused by allergy or sensitivity reactions because the symptoms are related to the tissues in which inflammatory chemicals are released. After exposure to a sensitizing agent, symptoms may manifest immediately or hours or days later.

Besides nasal congestion, symptoms include watery eyes, earache, blurred vision, tinnitus (buzzing or ringing of the ears), chronic cough, sore throat, and recurrent sinus infections. Congestion can move down to the chest, sometimes stimulating asthmatic spasms or even anaphylaxis (a severe and rapid allergic reaction involving many parts of the body, sometimes fatal).

> Any symptom can be caused by allergy or sensitivity
> reactions because the symptoms are related to the tissues
> in which inflammatory chemicals are released.

Allergic reactions on the outside of the body involve hives and other skin rashes, excessively dry skin, and brittle hair and nails. Urticaria (hives) occurs in the skin as welts. They appear swollen, raised, and red with different sizes and shapes. Atopic dermatitis (eczema) is an allergic inflammation of the skin, often beginning in infancy. The raised red eruptions form itchy, scaling crusts. Eczema often runs in families that have long histories of allergies, asthma, and hay fever.

Allergic rhinitis (hay fever) is an allergic inflammation of nasal mucous membranes. Here the mast cells release of inflammatory mediators causes patients to suffer from sneezing, a runny nose, and watery eyes. Many of these patients will also have asthma, sinusitis, and hives.

More difficult to pin down as allergy-related are gastrointestinal symptoms such as diarrhea, constipation, abdominal pain, and nausea, not to mention chronic fatigue and generalized joint or muscle pain. Still more elusive in terms of an allergy diagnosis are behavioral and psychological symptoms such as depression, hyperactivity, anxiety, aggressiveness, distractibility, irritability, slurred speech, and abnormal food cravings. You may notice that many of these symptoms also characterize ASD children, which is why they often respond to treatments for their allergies, once they have been identified.

DEFINITIONS

- **Allergy**: An exaggerated response of the immune system to specific substances that normally pose no threat to the human body, involving the elevation of specific antibodies due to antigen stimulus.

- **Sensitivity**: Any adverse reaction in the body that comes from exposure to a sensitizing agent in the environment. A sensitivity can involve antibodies and other immune processes. Food and chemical reactions are sensitivities.

- **Intolerance**: A reaction to food that does not involve the immune system. An intolerance presupposes the absence of a particular chemical or physiologic process needed to digest a food substance. For example, the lack of a digestive enzyme may result in a food intolerance

COMMON SYMPTOMS IN CHILDREN

Besides asthma symptoms, "hay fever" symptoms, and hives, what more specific symptoms in your child can tip you off about a potential allergy? Of course many of these symptoms can stem from other factors besides allergies, but when taken together with a suspected allergen or additional symptoms, you may logically determine that an allergy is at work.[1]

- Ticklish skin

- Excessive perspiration

- Unpleasant skin odor, especially of the feet

- Abnormally pale face

- Spaced-out facial expression

- Red tip of nose
- Red, itchy, watery eyes (frequently with bags or dark circles underneath)
- Red earlobes (one or both)
- Acute sensitivity to sounds
- Recurrent ear infections (associated nose, sinus, or lung infections)
- Red, circular, "rouge-like" cheek patches (especially in children ages one to four years)
- Rash around the mouth (from touching an allergenic substance such as toothpaste or chewing gum)
- Excessive drooling, unintentional spitting during conversation
- Canker sores in mouth
- "Patchy tongue," also known as "geographic tongue" (red, naked-looking "islands" surrounded by the normal pink color)
- Excessive thirst
- "Motor mouth" (i.e., hyperactivity expressed verbally)
- Repetitious whining (sometimes, if the repetition involves a food, the child is notifying the parent subconsciously that this food is the one that causes the allergic response)
- Stuttering, slurred speech
- Unusual sounds, such as mimicry of animal noises after exposure to allergenic substances
- Hoarse voice
- Cold hands and feet (can be related to problematic histamine levels in blood)

- Leg aches, restless legs

- Joint stiffness, like arthritis

- Lack of bladder control (like wheezing and spasms in the lungs, only in the bladder)

- Sleep problems

- Pimples on buttocks (or "scalded" buttocks on diapered infants)

- Red ring around anus, itchy genitals

- Obvious shifts or changes in ability to draw pictures or write words

Is reading these symptoms making you feel stuffy, itchy, and uncomfortable yourself? Even if you yourself do not suffer from any appreciable allergy symptoms (real or imagined), can you find your child's symptoms on this list? Have you noticed any patterns in the symptoms?

CAUSES OF ALLERGY AND SENSITIVITY

Research suggests that genetic factors predispose people to allergy and sensitivity, but no "allergy gene" has yet been found. We have to assume that early childhood practices lead to most allergies and sensitivities. Children should be the healthiest age group. They haven't been exposed to years of toxins, stress, and poor eating habits. Factors to consider include a toxic intrauterine environment, diet, breast- or bottle-feeding, too many vaccinations too early, and early introduction of solid foods.

Studies have shown about one-third of infants born to mothers with allergies will develop allergies as well. This may be because one of the immune mechanisms that lead to allergies is the transfer of IgG antibodies through the placenta from the mothers' blood into the fetal blood supply, which causes the developing baby to develop allergies to the same foods to which the mother is allergic. Even when the baby is breast-fed after birth (which reduces the risk of allergy development), the mother can transfer an allergic immune response passively before the baby's birth.

> Early childhood practices lead to most allergies and sensitivities.
> Children should be the healthiest age group.

As we discussed in chapter 2, early (and sometimes toxic) vaccinations also seem to be implicated in developing allergies. When young children are vaccinated against a virus, they never develop the disease, so their Th-1 cells do not need to respond strongly—which leads to increased Th-2 cell activity. Th-1 activity is cell-mediated immunity; the lymphocyte enters a virus-infected cell and kills the virus. Th-2 cell activity is antibody-mediated and does not happen inside an infected cell. As a result of what we call Th-2 "skewing," or predominance of antibody-mediated immunity, we get an allergic response.

OVERWHELMED IMMUNE SYSTEM

When any system reaches and exceeds its point of functional capacity, the system will malfunction. Where the immune system is concerned, we call this the "immune load."

Let's consider what your child's immune system has had to face. Besides environmental toxins such as agrochemicals and inhalant allergens, the likes of which never existed on the planet before, we add heavy metals from several sources and early-developing intestinal dysbiosis.

Once the capacity of your child's immune system was overwhelmed, most likely allergies developed at the slightest provocation (because of the Th-2 skewing that I mentioned above). This Th-2 skewing causes immune hyperactivity, which promotes more Th-2 skewing in a perpetuating cycle. The immune hyperactivity involves foods more than it would if the intestinal wall were intact and protected by predominantly healthy bacteria. If antibiotic overuse destroys them, overgrowth of harmful bacteria such as Candida albicans can increase gut wall permeability, allowing unwanted substances to migrate into the bloodstream where they may be identified as allergens and sensitization occurs.

This adds up to allergy and sensitivity. As we shall see, part of the healing will include reducing the immune load.

With healthy digestion and metabolism, food is not a sensitizing substance. The situation I have just described is essentially a delayed immune response. With careful observation and administration of a food elimination diet (see chapter 9), along with laboratory measurement of IgG and IgE antibodies, you can correlate your child's symptoms to exposure to certain foods.

Just as a healthy digestive system provides a protective barrier against the development of this delayed immune response, so healthy skin and mucous membranes provide protective barriers against potential allergens. Mucus traps foreign particles and removes them through coughing, sneezing, or normal ciliary action. Skin keeps foreign substances away from the circulatory system and the rest of the body. But if either a mucous membrane or part of the skin has been compromised by inflammation, the protection is compromised as well. Here again existing allergic reactions can give rise to more.

During early infancy children have an immature intestinal barrier to invasive substances. The helpful microflora has not yet increased sufficiently. Numerous variables at birth can impair microbial colonization (e.g., the degree of hygiene, the mode of delivery, the administration of antibiotics). This makes it impossible for many infant formulas as well as processed solid foods, cow's milk, wheat cereal, and protein to be digested properly.

HOW ENVIRONMENTAL TOXICITY
AFFECTS THE IMMUNE SYSTEM

Environmental toxicity renders the body's natural detoxification system very inefficient through overload.

The functional barrier systems of the skin, respiratory system, and intestine become overloaded leading to sensitization. The skin barrier keeps us safe from contactant (e.g., pollen) or injected (e.g., insect bite) antigens. The mucous membrane barrier consists of the respiratory system, the throat, nasal passages, and lungs. This natural barrier protects a person from inhaled substances. The gut barrier includes the stomach and intestines, and it wards off antigens and pathogens ingested primarily as food.

Our biological systems remain resilient only if they are capable of optimal self-defense via efficient detoxification (neutralizing external toxins that have gained entry into the body) and detoxication (neutralizing internal toxins derived from normal metabolic processes in the body). These processes can occur only with optimal nutrition; otherwise, toxins gain the upper hand and set in motion the various mechanisms that lead to sensitization and allergy.

When any of these barrier functions are broken down due to poor diet, toxin exposure, or bacterial overgrowth, foreign molecules are able to pass through the barrier and enter the bloodstream. Upon first exposure to a specific foreign molecule in the bloodstream (sensitization), the immune system determines whether the substance may be harmful to the body. If it finds it to be potentially dangerous, it records the antigen identification information in its cellular memory and begins the production of antibodies, which is specifically designed to deactivate the antigen. When the body is again exposed to the antigen, the immune system identifies the antigen and mobilizes the release of a preselected antibody, setting in motion a complex series of events involving many biochemicals.

These chemicals are what produce the inflammation and typical symptoms of an allergic response. The antibody most commonly involved in the allergic response to pollen and other aeroallergens is immunoglobulin E (IgE). The main types of immunoglobulins involved in the immune system's defense response to foreign substances are IgG, IgA, IgM, IgE, and mast cells, which are concentrated in the skin, nose, lungs, and GI tract. When an antibody senses an antigen, it triggers the mast cell to release histamine and two other chemicals. Both IgG and IgM antibodies neutralize bacteria, viruses, and toxins so that they can be destroyed by other immune cells. IgA antibodies in the gut mucous membranes neutralize antigens before they enter the bloodstream to trigger an allergic response.

An allergen (a substance provoking an allergy symptom) is very often a protein the body judges to be foreign and dangerous and thus attacks it. An allergen, by definition, stimulates the production of antibodies. Almost any agent can trigger allergic reactions; however, substances you inhale or ingest are the main allergens.

If toxic overload throws the immune system out of balance and chronic allergies develop, they perpetuate a heightened allergic reactivity, and the immune system becomes hyperactive. This can lead to autoimmune diseases.

The human body is a unit, and the various systems communicate

---

DEFINITIONS

- **Detoxification:** Neutralization and elimination of external toxins that have gained entry into the body.

- **Detoxication:** Neutralization and elimination of internal toxins derived from normal metabolic processes in the body.

- **IgE (immunoglobulin E):** Produced by plasma cells and lymphocytes, a protein that works by binding to allergens. It triggers the release of chemicals that can cause inflammation (i.e., an "allergic reaction").

- **IgG (immunoglobulin G):** A protein produced by plasma cells and lymphocytes, also known as gamma globulin; a major class of immunoglobulins that includes many of the antibodies that circulate in the blood.

- **IgM (immunoglobulin M):** An immunoglobulin that supplies "first-responder" antibodies that are replaced by other antibodies later in the immune response.

- **Histamine:** Substance released by mast cells when an allergen is encountered. Histamine increases the permeability of blood vessel walls and causes itching, hives, eye irritation, and sneezing in the person having the allergic reaction.

with one another. With regard to allergy, one can beget another (not necessarily of the same type). Inflammation from a food or inhalant allergy can render the immune system hypersensitive and hyperactive so that other substances can cause more inflammation at the slightest provocation. It becomes an endless cycle of inflammation throughout the body.

Widespread inflammation in the brain of an autistic child or the lungs of an asthmatic can be traced to earlier inflammation in the gut, and overall the inflammation increases as the digestive system, nervous system, and immune system communicate with one another.

IMMEDIATE HYPERSENSITIVITY (IGE-MEDIATED) ALLERGIES

Allergies that are IgE-mediated are the "classic" allergic conditions. The symptoms are readily visible; they are called "active" allergies or "true" allergies in conventional medical literature. IgE-mediated reactions occur minutes after exposure to an allergen, and they affect a relatively small proportion of all people who have reactions to foods.

> Widespread inflammation in the brain of an autistic child or the lungs of an asthmatic can be traced to earlier inflammation in the gut.

Let's say an individual has an allergy to the flowering plant known as goldenrod. Walking outside, the person breathes in the goldenrod pollen, and the person's immune system identifies it as a known allergen, signaling the production of IgE antibodies, which attach themselves to the surface of mast cells located in the respiratory and gastrointestinal systems. The IgE antibodies also attach to eosinophils, a type of white blood cell found in the bloodstream.

After a time this same individual breathes in more goldenrod pollen, which gets captured by attachment to the IgE antibody receptor site on the mast cells and eosinophil immune cells. These cells are then triggered to release inflammatory chemical mediators that are responsible for symptoms that vary according to the tissues in which they are found. A reaction in the mucous membranes of the nose results in swelling and increased secretion of mucus. In the lungs it results in difficulty breathing from contraction of the smooth muscles that line the bronchial tubes. The person's body is trying to neutralize and remove a foreign invader—the goldenrod pollen.

Food reactions, including both IgE allergies and IgG sensitivities, as well as intolerances (which are not caused by the immune system but rather by chemical reactions), are so widespread among 4-A kids as to be almost universal. I have yet to meet a 4-A child who does not struggle with one or more food reactions.

IGG SENSITIVITIES

Food sensitivities are far more common than IgE allergies. The most common foods that bring on these reactions are milk, wheat, egg, corn, and peanuts.

However, food allergies may be undiagnosed due to false negative reactions to skin and other IgE measurement tests, which cannot detect this allergic process, since it is IgG- and IgM-mediated. In a healthy immune

> **DEFINITION:**
>
> - Urticaria (hives): Occurs in the skin as welts. Lesions appear swollen, raised, and red with different sizes and shapes. The skin allows us to actually see the results of inflammatory mediators at work.
> - Sinusitis: Allergic inflammation of sinus cavities; sinus infection.
> - Eczema (atopic dermatitis): Allergic inflammation of the skin, often beginning in infancy, appearing after a baby stops breast feeding. This skin has a raised red eruption that forms scaling crusts with itching as a principle symptom. Eczema has a familial occurrence with long histories of allergies, asthma, and hay fever.
> - Allergic rhinitis (hay fever): Allergic inflammation of nasal mucous membranes. Here the mast cells release of inflammatory mediators causes patients to suffer from sneezing, runny nose, and watery eyes. Many of these patients will also have asthma, sinusitis, and hives.
> - Mast cells: Cells in connective tissue that release histamine and other inflammatory chemicals when injured in an allergic reaction.
> - Eosinophils: Are a type of white blood cell, part of the immune system, that contain particles filled with chemicals to conquer infections. The blood does not carry a large number of eosinophils unless your body needs to produce more of them in an allergic or inflammatory response, or in the case of parasitic infections.

system, immune cells neutralize the circulating immune complex that has been formed when an IgG antibody binds to foreign particles in the blood. But in a person with a compromised immune system, the circulating immune complex builds up to the point that it cannot be eliminated in the urine, and it ends up being deposited in tissues, causing inflammation. This process is implicated in the brain inflammation seen in autistic children as well as the lung inflammation seen in asthmatics. It should be considered a food allergy because it involves immunoglobulins and antibodies. And when the suspected foods are eliminated from the diet, the inflammation clears up accordingly.

Over eighty different medical conditions have been chemically associated with IgG food allergy reactions. These are delayed allergic or sensitivity reactions occurring seventy-two hours or more after exposure. The symptoms of these disorders, syndromes, or illnesses appear completely unrelated to allergies and can occur in any organ system. Allergic food reactions cause indigestion, heartburn, gas, and bloating. Food reactions give rise to hypoglycemia. The millions of patients with irritable bowel syndrome (IBS) should be directed to its primary cause: allergic food reactions. Studies have shown that pediatric migraine patients stopped having headaches when reactive foods were eliminated from their diets.

Food reactions starting in the gut disrupt insulin metabolism and contribute to inflammation of the pancreas in diabetics. Immune cells attacking beta cells in the pancreas have been found to cause type 1 diabetes (an autoimmune disease), which is increasing at an alarming rate. Does a surge of toxins in umbilical cord blood from the mother to the baby arrive in the developing baby's pancreas and alter the identity of the beta cells, rendering them foreign to the immune system so that it attacks and destroys them? Is it the aluminum found in vaccines given to very young infants triggering the toxic events in the pancreas? It is coincidental that the marked increase in incidence of type 1 diabetes coincides with the introduction of toxic vaccine programs (too many, too young, and too toxic)? Or that maternal diets during pregnancy include foods containing casein (milk protein) and gluten (grain protein) and foods high in nitrates (all of which have been associated with type 1 diabetes causality)?

INTOLERANCES

When we talk about a food "intolerance," the immune system is not involved. A food intolerance means that a person's body does not synthesize appropriate quantities of certain enzymes necessary to digest various foods. They are intolerant of that food, and cannot digest, metabolize, or assimilate it. Intolerance to a range of foods can cause unpleasant symptoms.

Lactase deficiency (a lack of the enzyme lactase, which digests lactose, or milk sugar) leads to lactose intolerance. Even if conventional IgE allergy tests are negative for a milk allergy, the intolerant patient will suffer from milk ingestion just the same. (While it is relatively easy for an allergist to test for inhalant IgE allergies, it is a longer process to determine a non-IgE reaction such as lactose intolerance.)

> When we talk about a food "intolerance," the immune system is not involved.

What happens in this kind of a non-antibody-mediated event? Since intolerances are distinguished from allergy/sensitivity in that the immune system is not involved (there is no antibody response), intolerances can come and go spontaneously; they are related to the individual's ability to metabolize substances. (By contrast, allergies and allergic sensitivities are consistent; your body will always make antibodies when challenged with an antigen.) Food intolerances are very common, especially intolerances to foods high in histamines (for example, spinach, tomatoes, fermented foods). When these foods are consumed, they can result in an inflammatory, pseudo-allergic response.

Chemical intolerance manifests with brain inflammation ("brain fog," depression, and fatigue), because pesticides in food, vehicle exhaust in the air, heavy metals in the water, and synthetic chemicals in cleaning products and building materials have accumulated in body fat instead of being eliminated. The composition of a person's brain is more than half fat.

Since allergies, sensitivities, and intolerances are rampant in the entire 4-A population, you can see why allergies have been granted a berth on the 4-A train. In fact, understanding the mechanisms of allergic responses, sensitivities, and intolerances is vital to the healing process for any of these other disorders. That is why I have given so much attention to nutritional strategies and other paths of healing that will help to straighten out the underlying causes of dysfunction.

HEALING

As I explained in chapter 3, an integrative approach to healing is the only one that will make significant progress against any part of the 4-A epidemics. As an integrative pediatrician with a special concern for children who suffer not only from allergies but also often from asthma, ADHD, and autism, my mission is to give my young patients their lives back to the fullest extent possible.

Toward that end and with the collaboration of parents, allergists, and other healing professionals, I apply a synergistic mix of four healing factors: nutrition, supplements, detoxification, and medications. As healing begins to take hold, the children themselves can better learn and cooperate with their own healing.

The principal medical professional member of the healing team must be well versed and experienced in integrative medicine in order to make the best choices for healing solutions, tailored to the unique needs of each child. Parents must get on board from the beginning, educating themselves, making necessary changes in the family diet and environment, keeping track of results day by day, and committing their resources to their child's fullest possible recovery.

With allergies and immune dysfunction as a particular focus, we need to listen to the "gut flora" experts such as Dr. Natasha Campbell-McBride of Cambridge, England, originator of the term GAPS for Gut and Psychology Syndrome and author of the book, *Gut and Psychology Syndrome: Natural Treatment for Autism, ADD, ADHD, Depression, Dyslexia, Dyspraxia, Schizophrenia*. Here she summarizes much of what I have put forward in this chapter:

> Well functioning gut flora is the right hand of our immune system. The beneficial bacteria in the gut ensure appropriate production of different immune cells, immunoglobulins and other parts of the immunity. But most importantly they keep the immune system in the right balance....
>
> These children commonly suffer from digestive problems, allergies, asthma and eczema. But apart from that in children and adults who then go on to develop neurological and psychiatric problems something even more terrible happens. Without control of the beneficial bacteria different opportunistic and pathogenic bacteria, viruses and fungi have a good chance to occupy large territories in the digestive tract and grow large colonies. Two particular groups which are most commonly found on testing are yeasts (including Candida species) and Clostridia family. These pathogenic microbes start digesting food in their own way producing large amounts of various toxic substances, which get absorbed into the blood stream, carried to the brain and cross the blood-brain barrier. The number and mixture of toxins can be very individual, causing different neurological and psychological symptoms. Due to the absence or greatly reduced numbers of beneficial bacteria in the gut flora, the person's digestive system instead of being

a source of nourishment becomes a major source of toxicity in the body.[2]

Though classic IgE-mediated allergies are part of the 4-A epidemic, far more of our autistic, ADHD, and asthmatic children are suffering from intolerances and disordered immune systems that can begin to heal and return to robust balance with the diligent efforts of their parents and dedicated integrative medical specialists.

SECTION III

HEALING THERAPIES FOR THE 4-A DISORDERS

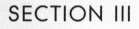

Chapter 8

Chapter 8

✠ ?! 𝄞 ✺

OVERVIEW OF THERAPIES

Marco's mother, Maria, arrived with him at my office for the first time when he was twenty-four months old. I could tell immediately after I introduced myself that she was desperately looking for help. How gratifying it was to see her anxious expression gradually change to a gentle smile of relief as I spoke.

As a doctor who has been entrusted with a gift, a life—in this case, little Marco—I open my mind, practice, and heart to join with both parent and child to tackle the job we have been given, and I respect the parent as a medical colleague and friend. Networking with other parents and compassionate doctors, listening and learning, watching Marco's reactions, assessing the next plan of action—all of it together comprises a holistic approach to healing.

"Marco is an individual with his own unique story, and he will be treated as an individual," I explained to Maria. "Marco's illness is a signal that changes must be made. Although genetic factors are important in an illness, they are hard to change. What can be changed is the *expression* of Marco's genetic information. We will discover ways to make complex genetic expressions change in order to undo the damage done by his environment. Marco was born with one or more genetic predispositions that make him susceptible to one or more types of environmental exposure. Today we will begin to figure it out and turn it around."

Maria had already filled out a chronological questionnaire about Marco's life, and I had reviewed it the evening before our appointment. Together we could now take a concentrated look at the time line of events leading to the present: (1) likely genetic predisposition, (2) possible exposure to toxins, including mercury, (3) administration of antibiotics in the first months of life, (4) consequent damage to Marco's gastrointestinal tract and its flora, (5) additional damage to his developing immune system, (6) live virus exposure via his first MMR vaccination at twelve months, (7) gastrointestinal, immunological, central nervous system signs and symptoms, and (8) laboratory evidence of inflammation and the spectrum disorder. Another lengthy questionnaire had documented Marco's symptoms and developmental problems.

> I realized that the holistic integrative model of care was my only logical choice for evaluating, diagnosing, treating, and monitoring these children's areas of need, and that it would be the only pathway for eventual (God willing) healing.

I reviewed with her the biochemistry of the metabolic problems that I felt were causing his disorder. We discussed a possible treatment plan, along with details of its implementation. I explained my interpretation of the outcomes of the treatments Maria had already obtained for her son. Finally, before interpreting the latest laboratory data, I examined Marco, who behaved as a perfect patient, and I told her how lovable he was.

We decided to start with a specific carbohydrate diet and a customized list of supplements. We also decided to address Marco's sleep problems and constipation with specific alternative therapies. I ordered additional laboratory studies for the present and three months from then.

Prior to beginning the specific carbohydrate diet, we decided to conduct a food allergen elimination. I started Marco on vitamin B_{12} and asked Maria to provide him with foods known to increase the body's production of glutathione (a list was given to her). I gave her some antifungal medication to treat Marco's GI yeast problem and told her that we could start other detox therapies within a month.

At the end of our lengthy appointment, I gave Maria my personal contact information and gave her some information about how to follow specific progress reports, contacting me every two weeks. After a prayer together, the appointment was concluded with a warm handshake.

INTEGRATIVE APPROACH TO HEALING THE 4-A DISORDERS

It has been twenty years now that I have been traveling the holistic integrative medicine highway, practicing systems medicine, integrating healing modalities, and treating each patient as a unique individual. I have attended numerous conferences, seminars, lectures, and courses of instruction in the integrative model. I have conducted informal clinical research with my patients and networked with many prominent figures also practicing this model: professors, clinicians, research scientists, authors and lecturers.

Early in my study of the 4-A epidemic the fact of its immense complexity struck me, and I realized that the holistic integrative model of care was my only logical choice for evaluating, diagnosing, treating, and monitoring these children's areas of need, and that it would be the only pathway for eventual (God willing) healing. Already I was open-minded about a wide range of treatments. I only needed to establish in my mind the essential importance of close collaboration and communication between me and the parents of my young 4-A patients.

COMBINING THERAPIES FOR HEALING

As I have mentioned more than once in this book, each child must receive a combination of therapies that has been tailored individually—after careful evaluation by an integrative physician who can best assess the many options and who knows how to combine them.

We must keep multiple, interdependent goals in view:

1. Detoxifying the child's systems

2. Eliminating further toxic exposure and accumulation

3. Healing the damaged systems using a variety of therapies

4. Restoring the fullest possible function to the immune system, the gastrointestinal system, and the nervous system

Every single child is different. Some, like Marco, come with hard-to-penetrate layers of 4-A dysfunction. Others may need only some nutritional "tweaking" to eliminate the aggravation of a single food allergy. But the initial evaluation must consider all of the elements of a complete healing program, which are, in brief, as follows.

Nutritional therapy

To start the nutritional component of therapy, we need to determine if the child has any food allergies, as well as food sensitivities and intolerances. After eliminating those particular foods from the child's diet, we need to take a look at other likely nutritional troublemakers. Children who react to gluten and casein must be sure to avoid wheat and dairy products and sometimes more. For some children it is also crucial to limit the foods that promote the growth of yeast.

More than one set of symptoms may indicate the limitation of carbohydrates as well. In any special diet only the most wholesome, organic, nutrient-dense foods should be supplied. This means eating only fruits and vegetables that have been grown without herbicides and pesticides and avoiding meats that have been treated with hormones, antibiotics, or arsenic. Most 4-A children should avoid eating tuna fish, a prime culprit in mercury contamination.

See chapter 9, "Healing Through Nutritional Therapy," for a much more in-depth look at the nutritional component of 4-A healing.

Supplemental therapy

I always start children off with nutrient-dense supplements that are also rich in antioxidants, including a specific whole-food concentrate of fruits and vegetables. (See Appendix D.) Their systems may have been depleted and degraded to the point that they cannot absorb enough nutrients from food alone, especially while we are learning which foods need to be eliminated and while we are still modifying their food preferences. Particular and individualized supplements (vitamins, enzymes, and minerals) are given, based on deficiencies indicated by laboratory studies.

Always I find that we need to supplement with probiotics in order to restore the proper bacterial flora in the child's gut and to help control yeast overgrowth. In addition I recommend supplements that can help the child's body to detoxify various systems (GI, nervous, etc.) and to kill the bacteria, funguses, and sometimes parasites that have attacked the child's gastrointestinal system. Often additional supplements help improve energy, cognition, and behavior.

You can read more about my approach to the supplemental side of 4-A therapy in chapter 10, as well as in some of the disorder-specific aspects in Appendixes A, B, and C.

Detoxification therapy

Detoxification means getting rid of the toxic overload in a child's body—and keeping it out. In chapter 11, "Healing Through Detoxification Therapy," I have detailed my typical detox "prescriptions." Some are as commonsense as drinking plenty of clean water, while others are as unusual as glutathione skin gel. (Glutathione is a powerful antioxidant, which is often low in 4-A children.) Children's natural detoxification chemistry can be helped by supplementary magnesium, niacin, and vitamin B_6 (sometimes made available via foods, not always via oral supplements).

Chelation therapy, which is an FDA-approved procedure that can be used to remove heavy metals such as mercury and lead from a child's system, has helped many children recover. Eliminating sources of toxins may mean the removal of amalgam dental fillings or moving to a different house or neighborhood. It definitely includes the avoidance of food additives such as dyes, artificial sweeteners, preservatives, MSG, hormones, and antibiotics. Often, for the sake of keeping toxic buildup at bay, we need to limit casein and gluten as well.

Medication therapy

Especially for some of the 4-A disorders, prescription medicines are an important part of the healing process. Some of them accomplish things that no natural supplement or procedure can supply, such as the bronchodilation that can be a literal lifesaver for an asthmatic child.

We also need to resort to various anti-inflammatories, antibiotics, antifungals, and antivirals in our fight against a multifaceted enemy. Certain children need psychoactive medications too, and allergic reactions may compel the use of antihistamines.

Chapter 12 contains a helpful overview of the most common medications that may help your own child.

Please read on through the next pages, picking out of the next four chapters the most useful information for your own child. As I cannot reiterate too often, each child is completely unique, and while I can certainly help you recognize unhealthy patterns and recommend their likely remedies, you and your integrative physician will need to test out various approaches to see what works.

The most important healing therapy of all is the one that has brought you this far and that will take you the distance—*love*.

Without the unconditional, unflagging love of mom and/or dad, your child cannot make headway against so many invisible adversaries at the same time. I am standing right beside you, supplying solid information and tangible hope.

Chapter 9

HEALING THROUGH NUTRITIONAL THERAPY

Handsome seventeen-year-old Cory was diagnosed with ASD at age three, after losing one developmental milestone after another. ADHD was diagnosed when he was six. Anxiety and panic attacks began when he was ten years old, and we realized we needed to find a treatment that went beyond learning and speech therapy, sensory integration and auditory training, all of which had helped initially. To help with his food allergies and sensitivities, we started him on the gluten-free/casein-free (GF/CF) diet, and he followed it for seven years. It helped, but eventually the same old problems recurred. Finally Cory made tremendous progress once we started him on the specific carbohydrate diet (SCD). Things just started to click. His friends comment often on his new, relaxed demeanor. His new diet seems to be linked to his increased language, socialization, focus, and academic success. After living through the horror of an immune and digestive system plagued by food sensitivities, recurrent diarrhea, constipation, and yeast infections, not to mention all the symptoms of the autism-ADD spectrum, he is now speaking hopefully about his future. He is also enjoying some foods he hasn't had for years. Cory is a success story, and I believe he will continue to be.

"IT ALL STARTS IN THE GUT"

Our children's nutrition is so important to their healing that I focus on it as early as possible and try to be as careful as possible. Their nutritional deficits are among the principal causes of their difficulties, and therefore nutritional therapy needs to become a major factor in the healing of the 4-A disorders.

> The multitude of 4-A symptoms involving all systems result from three types of food reactions: allergies, sensitivities, or intolerances.

Just as no 4-A patient is identical to any other, no single diet will heal all 4-A patients. Still we have zeroed in on several specific diets as good starting places, and we individualize them for each child. This chapter will provide you with an overview both of your child's metabolic problems and of how you can become well-equipped to use the most powerful medicine that will heal them: food.

Every doctor and parent who is caring for a child on the 4-A spectrum must be guided by the basic premise: "It all starts in the gut."

The truth is that the multitude of 4-A symptoms involving all systems result from three types of food reactions: allergies, sensitivities, or intolerances. Autistic and ADHD patients, as well as severe asthmatics, can attest to the fact that specific dietary restrictions have reduced their pain and suffering, relieved their breathing difficulty, and made it easier to learn and perform socially.

Naturally many young autistic patients cannot tell us how they feel. But their parents can see their silent suffering, and they can testify to how dietary changes have improved their family life. Sometimes the improvements are so dramatic and obvious that nobody needs to be told about them.

The fact is that peer-reviewed studies and many case studies have situated dietary intervention as a primary therapy for 4-A kids. If nothing else, gut issues have proven to complicate spectrum kids' symptoms. As has been shown in multiple studies, these children have skewed immune responses to the proteins in wheat, milk, and soy. Two of these partially digested proteins (more about them later) are known as gluteomorphine and casomorphine, and they are structurally similar to morphine, as you can tell by the "morphine" in their names. They affect opioid receptors in a child's brain, which may explain autistic symptoms such as sensory irregularities and stimming.

Dr. Timothy Buie, a Harvard pediatric gastroenterologist, has proven, through endoscopies and biopsies of hundreds of autistic children, that they all have chronic inflammation of the digestive tract along with enzyme deficiencies.[1] These children have faulty carbohydrate digestion and malabsorption. This explains the frequency of gastrointestinal symptoms such as pain and bloating, their allergic responses to foods, and their many vitamin and mineral deficiencies.

Only informed dietary intervention and change can begin to lead to healing. In this chapter I will introduce you to the following diets:

1. The gluten-free/casein-free (GF/CF) diet

2. Elimination diets

3. The anti-yeast diet

4. The anti-hypoglycemia diet

5. The specific carbohydrate diet (SCD)

6. The low oxalate diet

HOW ARE FOODS ABSORBED—OR NOT?

To understand the reasons for undertaking specific diets, we need to review how foods are absorbed in the digestive tract. This information will help us to better understand the reasons for food restrictions and recommendations.

The wall of the small intestine looks like velvet because it is lined with villi (little protrusions) that are composed of enterocytes—the cells that absorb food and pass it into the blood circulation to nourish our bodies. Enterocytes have a short life cycle, but they are constantly renewed. Their renewal is ruled by the beneficial bacteria that live on them and control enterocyte health and proper functioning. If the beneficial bacteria are missing or insufficient, leaving the absorptive surfaces of the villi covered with pathogenic, opportunistic microbes, the enterocytes cannot perform their job of absorbing food.

Monosaccharides (simple sugars, including glucose, fructose, and galactose) are the tiny molecules that comprise all carbohydrates. Monosaccharides can easily be absorbed through enterocytes into the bloodstream without the aid of other digestive processes. Fruits, vegetables, honey, and dairy products are the major sources of these monosaccharides.

Disaccharides ("di-" meaning two and "saccharide" meaning sugar molecules) are formed when two monosaccharides are joined together. For example: milk sugar (lactose) is composed of glucose and galactose, and the sugar from sugar cane and sugar beets (sucrose) is composed of glucose and fructose. Another disaccharide is maltose, which derives from starch (grains and starchy vegetables) in the diet.

The tiny hairs on the surface of enterocytes (microvilli) produce enzymes that break down disaccharides into monosaccharides to be absorbed. Here is where children with digestive disorders have their major problem. Enzyme-deficient enterocytes cannot break down disaccharides. As a consequence they remain in the gut where opportunistic microbes (bacteria and

DEFINITIONS

- Enterocytes: Specialized cells in the small intestine that absorb nutrients, electrolytes, and water.
- Carbohydrates: Mainly sugars and starches, sources of calories (energy) that come in simple forms (sugars) and complex forms (starches and fiber), which are broken down in the body into the simple sugar glucose. Carbohydrates are classified into mono-, di-, tri-, poly-, and heterosaccharides. The most basic and smallest carbohydrates are the monosaccharides.
- Disaccharides: A class of sugars (including sucrose and lactose) that yield two monosaccharide molecules.
- Monosaccharides: Simple sugars, including glucose, fructose, and galactose, that cannot be broken down further into other sugars.

funguses such as Candida) use them as food. This is why we place dietary restrictions on foods that yield disaccharides and why we do what we can to promote the repopulation of beneficial bacteria within the child's intestines.

Then we must consider the proteins that are initially broken down into peptides by the stomach and duodenal enzymes. Proteins consist of amino acids, and these peptides consist of amino acid chains that must be broken down to single amino acids by the microvilli of enterocytes in order to be absorbed. If enterocytes malfunction, as described, partially digested peptides are absorbed through a damaged gut wall (in particular, gluten from grains and casein from milk).

Meat, fish, and eggs are very digestible sources of protein, and fats are easily absorbed in a healthy gut. However, along with abnormal gut flora and inflammation of the gut wall comes an excessive amount of mucus production, which coats food particles. This prevents bile and enzymes from digesting the fats, and it can result in deficiencies of fat-soluble vitamins A, D, K, and E.

GLUTEN-FREE/CASEIN-FREE DIET

Because of the distress in their digestive tracts, most autistic kids, ADHD kids, and severe asthmatics, including all severely allergic children, will benefit from a diet that is strictly free of gluten (grains) and dairy (casein). The removal of these foods provides the foundation of dietary interventions in the 4-A disorders. Additional changes will always be needed for more complete improvement, but the standard initial dietary intervention is the gluten-free/casein-free (GF/CF) diet.

No single diet solves everything or applies across the board to many children. Yet the GF/CF diet shows the most promising results. Here's why:

> As long ago as 1971, researcher M. S. Goodwin documented abnormal brain responses to gluten. A decade

later, other researchers showed that children who maintained a gluten-free, casein-free diet showed improved cognition, language and behavior. It's now believed that certain peptides (amino acid chains) from gluten and casein can bind to opioid receptors in the brain, causing a powerful effect on behavior. Symptoms include "zoning out," aggression, self-abuse and constipation or diarrhea. These peptides appear to cause trouble for ASD [autism spectrum disorder] kids because of improper digestion and gut inflammation, common problems in this population....

The Autism Research Institute of San Diego tracks the efficacy of many treatments. Over 60 percent of its respondents report improvement from dietary intervention. TACA, a California support group, reported a better than 80 percent positive response from the diet, based on a survey it conducted of over 14,000 families. For some children, improvement is slight. For others, it is significant.[2]

As a protein, gluten requires a particular enzyme, DPP4, to break it down successfully within the human body. This enzyme is also involved in the digestion of milk and milk products, all of which contain casein. In children and adults in whom DPP4 does not function fully, the gluten and the casein do not get fully broken down. The result is peptides (partial proteins) that mimic the chemical composition of opiates or endorphins and cause similar feelings to occur when they reach the brain. The pleasure (spaciness and sense of intoxication) that this brings makes it very hard for kids to give up gluten. In fact, often they crave processed carbohydrates, the very foods that feed the pathogens in their gut. In addition one researcher has discovered that these peptides seem to interfere with the methylation process necessary for the body to detoxify itself.

The typical pattern of autistic-ADHD development includes the fact that within the first two years of life, the child limits his or her diet to dairy products, processed carbohydrates (breads, cakes, cookies, chips, cereals, pasta), and sugar. The pathogenic flora in their gastrointestinal systems love it, but nobody else does because of the plethora of troublesome symptoms that result. Nevertheless the kids themselves certainly don't want to change their food preferences and accept other foods.

Not all gluten-free and casein-free foods are the same. Since the GF/CF diet has become better known, companies have begun marketing prepared foods that may well be gluten- and casein-free—but they are full of sugar and altered fats and proteins. Spectrum children should not have these foods. Their gut dysbiosis will not be alleviated in the least, and their systems will not be healed. Learn what you are avoiding, and learn to read the labels; many gluten-free breads, crackers, pastas, and baking products are available from reputable companies.

> **DEFINITIONS**
>
> - Gluten: A protein with sticky qualities that comes from the outer endosperm of wheat seeds and related grains.
> - Casein: The most common protein found in milk.

Where do gluten and casein come from?

The kernels (seeds) of whole grains have three layers: (1) the outer bran layer, (2) the middle endosperm, and (3) the inner germ. Gluten is found in the middle, starchy layer, the endosperm. When grains are processed, only the endosperm remains. This is true for all varieties of wheat, including durum, einkorn, emmer, faro, kamut, and spelt, and also for barley, rye, and some oats. Also included is triticale, which is a hybrid of rye and wheat.

Casein is the most common protein found in milk, and therefore it can be found in all milk products.

How to choose the right foods and beverages

Foods labeled "wheat-free" are not necessarily gluten-free. You will need to become familiar with a complete list of the gluten- and casein-containing foods that your child will need to avoid in order to achieve success, as well as a list of gluten- and casein-free foods.[3]

Children must gradually become accustomed to meat, fish, and chicken that is simply broiled or baked. If they insist on breaded nuggets, breading can be prepared with acceptable flours or ground nuts. Parents must learn to be careful of hidden sources of gluten, such as the coating on commercially dried fruits. Gluten-containing breads, cakes, cookies, bagels, muffins, and snacks must be avoided, substituting gluten-free options when possible.

> Foods labeled "wheat-free" are not necessarily gluten-free, and foods labeled "dairy-free" are not necessarily casein-free.

Here are some partial food lists to give you the gist of the diet. (You will need to obtain complete advice from your integrative physician or a diet specialist whom he recommends to you.)

BASIC LIST OF FOODS ALLOWED ON THE GF/CF DIET

(This list must be modified to accommodate specific allergies and food sensitivities.)

- Almond milk and other nut milks
- Amaranth
- Beans and legumes (prepared from dry or unseasoned canned)
- Beef
- Buckwheat
- Chicken
- Coconut milk
- Corn flour
- Eggs
- Fish
- Fruits (all plain fresh or frozen, most canned, avoid dried)
- Fruit juices (plain)
- Lamb

- Meats (fresh or frozen, plain)
- Millet
- Nuts (all types, unflavored)
- Oats, if gluten-free
- Oils (all types)
- Quinoa
- Rice
- Rice milk
- Potatoes (fresh, plain)
- Seeds (all types)
- Shellfish
- Soy milk
- Turkey
- Vegetables (all unprocessed)

BASIC LIST OF FOODS TO AVOID

- Baby foods (prepackaged)
- Baked goods (bagels, biscuits, bread, bread crumbs, bread stuffing, cake, chow mein noodles, cookies, crackers, croissants, croutons, doughnuts, ice cream cones, muffins, pancakes, pastry, pies, pita bread, pizza, pretzels, rolls, tortillas, waffles, etc.)
- Barley, barley grass
- Beverage mixes
- Bologna
- Bouillon, instant
- Bran (except rice)
- Brewers yeast
- Broth, prepackaged
- Bulgur
- Butter
- Candy (most)
- Cereals (most)

- Cheeses
- Chicken nuggets (and any breaded meat or fish)
- Cold cuts
- Couscous
- Cream sauces
- Durum wheat
- Farina
- Flour
- Custard, pudding
- Gum (most)
- Hot dogs
- Ice cream, ice milk
- Kasha
- Kefir
- Marzipan
- Mashed potatoes
- Matzo semolina
- Milk (all types, from animal sources)
- Milk chocolate
- Muesli
- Nougat
- Pasta, noodles, macaroni, spaghetti
- Potato chips
- Salad dressings (creamy or commercially prepared)
- Sausage
- Semolina
- Sour cream
- Sprouted wheat or barley
- Tabbouleh
- Teriyaki sauce
- Triticale
- Rye
- Salad dressing (creamed, commercially prepared)

- Soy sauce
- Syrups
- Vegetables in sauces
- Wheat germ
- Wheat grass
- Yogurt
- Zwieback

You would be surprised at the hiding places of gluten and casein in prepackaged foods. For example, canned fish and prepared rice products may contain milk protein. Learn to read and understand the fine print on food labels, and recheck them each time you purchase the item because manufacturers can change ingredients. Package banners such as "dairy free," and "nondairy" do not mean casein-free, but only that the package contains less than 0.5 percent milk by weight—which translates into as much casein as whole milk.

It is hard for kids to give up the major food categories that make up the American diet. Often parents who report no improvement with the GF/CF diet are inadvertently feeding their children foods with hidden gluten and/or casein.

Here are some of the hidden sources of gluten and casein in common foods:

HIDDEN SOURCES OF GLUTEN AND/OR CASEIN

- Baking powder
- Cocoa
- Curry powder

Food items containing any of the following:

- "Binders"
- Caramel color
- Cereal binding
- Dextrimaltose

- "Edible starch"
- "Emulsifiers"
- "Filler"
- Hydrolized plant/vegetable/wheat starch, protein
- Malt
- Modified food starch
- "Natural flavor"
- Sodium caseinate
- "Stabilizer"
- Textured vegetable protein (TVP)
- Vegetable starch
- Wheat flour lipids
- Whey
- Fruit pie fillings
- Gravy
- Gummed envelopes or labels
- Margarine
- Mayonnaise
- Sandwich spreads
- Soups, canned
- Spam
- Spice mixtures (read ingredients)
- Vinegar

Cravings and symptoms

To begin dietary interventions, the child's food preferences must be determined accurately, since foods that are craved are usually problematic (and you will find that they are usually dairy- and wheat-based foods and sugar). Observe the child's symptoms carefully and document them. Note the child's behavior and appearance. For example, you may observe irritability, fatigue, anger, hyperactivity, inability to concentrate, or difficulty remembering. You may note puffiness under the eyes, dark eye circles, a top-of-the-nose wrinkle from upward nose-rubbing, bright red earlobes, abnormally rosy cheeks, a spacey expression, a tongue that looks like a map ("geographic tongue"), or pimples on the buttocks. You may be able to see that these symptoms seem to be connected with eating particular foods.

In a food diary document food lists and changes you observe after a food is eaten. Besides observations of behavior and appearance, have your child print letters or draw pictures before and after a food is eaten. Proceed with extra caution if a food causes wheezing problems in your asthmatic child. This food diary can be an important tool, in that it can reveal delayed food reactions, some of which can manifest in distant organ systems.

Give yourself about three months to try this diet. Within the first three weeks remove all dairy and gluten from the diet. You can retain sugar and starchy foods temporarily to help reduce withdrawal symptoms from the dairy and gluten restriction. But sugar and starchy foods must be eliminated as soon as possible, along with corn and soy, since most 4-A children have food reactions to not only dairy and gluten but also to sugar, starchy foods, corn, and soy. I advise that the elimination of these foods occur in a relatively rapid fashion, in less than forty days. If your child remains symptomatic during the dairy and gluten restriction, it could indicate a reaction to sugar, corn, or soy if these have not been eliminated from the diet.

The most important foods to substitute are fresh fruits and vegetables, raw or steamed. If your child dislikes these choices, you might try blenderized versions. You might also supplement with a whole-food concentrate and a probiotic to provide some of the benefits your child has been missing. (See Appendix D.)

Carefully read labels of everything your child eats or drinks. Besides becoming aware of the many ingredients in a processed food, you want to make sure that it is free of additives. If you are suspicious of a food, start with tiny amounts and increase gradually during the day.

Evaluating the results

How long should you keep your child on the GF/CF diet? You should be able to tell within a few weeks if casein restrictions are helping, and within about three months regarding gluten restrictions. If your child does have a problem with one or both, things should improve noticeably when they are eliminated. If nothing improves, feel free to abandon the trial. Natural healing takes time, which is why three months may be required to give the diet a fair trial.

Before you decide whether or not to continue with the GF/CF diet, you may need to press through "withdrawal" symptoms from gluten and casein. In other words your child's symptoms may worsen at first. If, however, your child happens to have a classic IgE allergy to wheat or another gluten-containing grain, you may notice almost immediate improvement.

Well into the trial, an IgG multiple food allergy blood test could uncover other problematic foods, along with an IgE food and environmental allergy blood test. A comprehensive digestive stool analysis could screen for parasites and organic acid urine analysis for other gut problems.

If no changes are noted after three weeks on a GF/CF diet, remember to eliminate the other foods that these children typically cannot process. This includes corn, starchy vegetables, soy, and the remaining complex carbohydrates. More than 60 percent of 4-A children will improve on this diet, which is why it has become the single most popular dietary intervention.

Positive outcomes can include improved health, healthy functioning digestive and pulmonary systems, and improved cognitive and learning abilities. Your child will begin to respond to feelings in on appropriate manner. Other improvements may include changes in language skills, mood disorders, hyperactive behavior, eczema, insomnia, fatigue, bloating, and food cravings. Carefully monitored dietary changes can bring about striking improvements in as short a time as two weeks.

Once your child's gut heals, some of the eliminated foods may be reintroduced successfully. Some children will need to follow this diet, at least in a modified form, for the rest of their lives. But they will be in good company, because so many other children and adults in the Western world have adopted this diet as well. Support groups and food choices abound, and following these dietary restrictions may be one of the best things that ever happened for these 4-A children.

Dangerous food additives

MSG (monosodium glutamate) is derived from glutamate, a neurotransmitter. It can cause immune-mediated reactions (IgE, IgG), but mainly intolerance reactions occur. Glutamate is a sodium salt of glutamic acids; it is an amino acid that occurs naturally in many foods, where it gets broken down slowly during digestion to prevent the surges that are associated with pure processed additive MSG.

Processed MSG is added as a ubiquitous flavor enhancer to almost every canned, packaged, or otherwise processed food sold in stores. Because it fools the brain into thinking something tastes better than it actually does, manufacturers may use it in lieu of quality ingredients.

Experimental studies have shown that MSG kills neurons (nerve cells) by exciting them to death. This is called excitotoxicity. After a food containing glutamate is digested, glutamate levels in the blood are elevated. Our blood-brain barrier was designed to prevent this glutamate from entering the brain and setting off destructive excitotoxicity, but in autism and ADHD, the blood-brain barrier has become defective.

Aspartame and carrageenan fall into the same category; they should be avoided by 4-A children because of their excitotoxic properties and for their tendency to cause inflammation and stimulate the growth of cancerous cells. Excitotoxins and their metabolites manifest with symptoms of hyperactivity and behavioral problems. Other food additives to avoid include EDTA, sulfites, nitrates, dyes, and bromates.

Careful scrutiny is needed to determine if a child is reacting to a food or a food additive. Avoiding all processed foods is a step in the right direction.

ELIMINATION DIETS

I'm sure that it is becoming increasingly evident that food can inter-fere with how your child performs in school or at home. Since allergies are one of the 4-A disorders, we need to include a diet that will help detect food allergies

Your child may already have had skin tests to detect IgE anti-bodies for nonfood allergies such as pollen. But food allergies, unless they are exceptionally severe and point clearly to a particular food item, are harder to detect. Food intolerances (not the same as a full-blown allergy) are elusive because they do not involve the immune system, so the ordinary lab tests will not work for them. You know your child's insides are inflamed and messed up, but you have no clue about the role of each particular food in the overall picture.

Fortunately, a preferred way to detect food allergies, sensitivities, and intolerances involves no medical fees at all, because it's a matter of food choices. Quite literally by a process of elimination you will be able to identify which foods are perpetuating your child's problems.

You can approach this process of elimination one food at a time (the single food elimination diet) or you can try eliminating several foods at a time (the multiple foods elimination diet).

Elimination diet for a single food (a diagnostic diet)

You might want to start with a frequently eaten food. For ten days have your child stop eating that food in every form. After twelve days if the symptoms have gone away, offer the food again. If the symptoms return, you will know your child has a food sensitivity.

This diet is fairly simple to keep track of. It gives you definite answers, as long as you adhere to strict parameters. Not only should you police your child's diet consistently for the ten- to twelve-day period, you should reintroduce the food all by itself after a four-hour fast. Symptoms may return from one hour after consumption to a few days after repeated samplings.

The major disadvantage of this diet is that it's slow going. Once or twice a month you will be able to check off one or two more foods. In the meantime life hurtles along with its many challenges.

Elimination diet for multiple foods (a diagnostic diet)

If you want to undertake an elimination diet for multiple foods at the same time, start by eliminating all of the foods that most commonly cause allergies. This will include all foods that contain wheat, eggs, corn, dairy products, chocolate (cocoa or cola), peas, peanut butter, citrus fruits, food coloring, food additives, and preservatives.

"Wait!" you say. "What can I feed my child? That's almost everything!" No it's not. For your reference here is a chart of allowed and forbidden foods:[4]

ALLOWED CEREALS	FORBIDDEN CEREALS
Rice puffs only	Wheat flour–containing foods
Oatmeal (with honey only)	Corn
Barley	Cereal mixtures (granola)
ALLOWED FRUITS	**FORBIDDEN FRUITS**
Fresh fruits, except citrus	Citrus fruit (fresh, frozen, canned)
Canned fruits (in own juice)	
ALLOWED VEGETABLES	**FORBIDDEN VEGETABLES**
All other fresh vegetables	Corn, peas, mixed vegetables
Potatoes	
ALLOWED MEATS	**FORBIDDEN MEATS**
Chicken, turkey	Bacon, ham
Beef, veal	Lunch meat, wieners
Pork	Artificially colored meats
Lamb	Breaded or stuffed meats
Fish	

ALLOWED BEVERAGES	FORBIDDEN BEVERAGES
Water	Milk in any form
Grape juice, bottle, natural	Sodas
Apple juice, frozen, natural	Kool-Aid
ALLOWED SNACKS	**FORBIDDEN SNACKS**
Potato chips, natural	Corn chips
Ry-Krisp	Anything chocolate or cocoa
Raisins (unsulfured)	Hard candy
	Ice cream, sherbet
ALLOWED MISCELLANEOUS	**FORBIDDEN MISCELLANEOUS**
Pure honey	Sugar (all forms)
Homemade vinaigrette	Peanut butter, peanuts
Sea salt	Eggs
Pepper	Sorbitol (corn)
Homemade soup	Canned soups
	Bread and baked goods
	Jelly, jam, Jell-O
	Margarine (unless no dyes, corn)
	Cheese

You will need to keep your child on this diet for a little over two weeks. For the first seven days, adhere strictly to the guidelines. Then begin to reintroduce the foods, one at a time, keeping track of your child's symptoms. (If you already know that one of these categories causes a problem for your child, don't bother to reintroduce that one.) Allergist Dr. Doris Rapp, whose recommendations I follow, recommends that you reintroduce the foods in the following order: day 8: milk; day 9: wheat; day 10: sugar; day 11: eggs; day 12: cocoa; day 13:

food coloring; day 14: corn; day 15: preservatives; day 16: citrus; day 17: peanut butter.

As you reintroduce various foods, you will want to write down what happens. Do not rely on your memory, because you will be dealing with so many variables. Offer the food multiple times during the day, preferably by itself, starting with a very small amount (as little as a teaspoon), and doubling the amount every few hours so that by the end of the day a normal amount will have been consumed. Pay attention to your child's reactions within an hour of eating the food each time. Do any of his or her symptoms return? Do they return after several "doses" of the test food? If not, your child is probably not sensitive to that type of food, and it can be added back with the "safe" foods. If any of the foods causes serious symptoms, eliminate it immediately and seek the advice of your doctor.

The next day test another one of the foods that you had eliminated during the first phase of the diet. In between the times when you give your child the test food, you may give any of the safe foods; this diet does not require your child to live on one item to the exclusion of the others. You are only trying to isolate the food items that make trouble for your child. If your child attends school, you can reintroduce the foods starting with the after-school snack.

Within two weeks if your child's symptoms disappear, you will have discovered which foods have been causing distress for such a long time.

Parents observe results

As I mentioned, you will need to keep a written record of the results of your testing. This is an observation (visual, auditory, or anecdotal) that compares five variables before and ten to sixty minutes after an exposure to a food.

Dr. Rapp has narrowed down the pertinent observations to what she calls The Big Five:[5]

1. How does my child feel/behave? (Is there a characteristic change in how your child felt, acted, or behaved?)

2. How does my child look? (Do you see red earlobes,
   dark eye circles, nose rubbing, throat clearing, wiggly
   legs, lip licking, itchy skin?)

3. Is there handwriting or drawing change? (Have your
   child write or draw the same thing before and after
   the food is ingested. Does the handwriting or drawing
   match, or does it turn out two different ways?)

4. Is there a breathing problem? (Does breathing
   become labored, wheezy, congested?)

5. Is there a change in the pulse rate? (Take your child's
   pulse before and after the food is ingested. Does it
   become irregular or too fast? This could mean that
   the body has gone into a state of alarm.)

Other reactions such as eczema, bed-wetting, and GI tract problems can occur hours later. It should go without saying that you
should not bother to test any food to which your child has had a severe
allergic reaction in the past.

The elimination diet for multiple foods is meant to be a temporary
one—three weeks at most. It is a diagnostic test only. Do not continue
it indefinitely because of the risk of malnourishment.

ANTI-YEAST DIET

Too many 4-A children suffer endlessly from yeast (or Candida) overgrowth. You will have noticed already that I mention it often as I
describe the constellation of these kids' symptoms. As you are narrowing down your own child's acceptable food choices, this is one
more consideration for your concern.

Candida albicans is a type of fungus that thrives under certain
conditions in the human body. Unfortunately those conditions are all

too often present in the immune-compromised little bodies of our 4-A children. In addition to having unbalanced digestive systems, they often require antibiotics to fight bacterial infections. Antibiotics wipe out the "good bacteria" in the gut as well as the harmful ones, further challenging the child's system. In the gut Candida proliferates from its harmless one-cell state into an active invasive state, growing long stringy roots that penetrate the gut wall and weaken the space between the enterocytes, causing a "leaky gut" to develop. This sort of growth also results in the production of a whole host of toxic substances as well. These microscopic holes in the gut wall allow undigested food particles to enter the bloodstream, causing damage to the immune and nervous systems.

How can you tell if your child's symptoms stem from a yeast overgrowth (also called a yeast infection) or from the many other factors? One surefire sign that it's yeast is the tongue and mouth infection known as thrush. Take a look inside your child's mouth. Do you see whitish patches on the tongue or moist skin? Look no farther; it's yeast.

Even if you do not see signs of thrush, a yeast overgrowth can be present. What you thought was "just diaper rash" was probably yeast overgrowth, especially if you can't get rid of it. Certainly you should suspect yeast as the culprit if your son has "jock itch," or if your daughter has vaginal infections with white mucus. Other symptoms can be attributed to yeast overgrowth, but they overlap significantly with 4-A symptoms with which you are already familiar, such as restlessness, difficulty sleeping, cognitive problems, water retention, and more.

If your child is already on the GF/CF diet, you will have fewer changes to make to help conquer the yeast overgrowth. That's because many of the yeast-promoting foods are already disallowed on the GF/CF diet, such as breads and other baked goods (because they often contain yeast as a leavening agent and because they are sweet) and casein-containing foods such as cheese (Roquefort and similar cheeses being targeted in the anti-yeast diet because they sport mold as part of the taste). Sugar stimulates the yeast overgrowth, so your child should not eat or drink any sweetened item, including honey, fruit juices, or dried fruits.

To be on the safe side on the anti-yeast diet, you should add these types of items to your "no-no" list: catsup, pickles, olives, sauerkraut, mustard, vinegar, cider, and mushrooms (a fungus itself). Good-bye, hot dogs! (You already eliminated the buns and the dogs, and now you have eliminated all the condiments.)

As symptoms disappear, you can reintroduce some of the foods that are not limited by your other dietary measures.

ANTI-HYPOGLYCEMIA DIET

All 4-A kids have episodes of hypoglycemia, or low blood sugar. It is inordinately common in environmentally ill, allergic children. Signs and symptoms of hypoglycemia include headache, bad mood, tantrums, aggression, general fatigue, drowsiness, whining, shaking, irritability, anger, hyperactivity, insomnia, craving for sweet/starchy foods, night sweats and profuse perspiration, expressive language problems, poor cognition, and inattentiveness. This list, you probably noted as you read it, also describes an ADHD or autistic child. In fact, hypoglycemic children have been misdiagnosed with ADHD and autism. These symptoms are also found in patients with Candida (yeast) overgrowth and food reactions (allergy sensitivities or intolerance).

Needless to say, parents and integrative physicians who are treating children with ADHD and autism (children who are also burdened with environmental toxicity and nutritional deficiencies) acquire a full appreciation for this complex combination of symptoms.

Hypoglycemic children who have a food sensitivity have symptoms before they eat from low blood sugar and after they eat because of the food allergy. Their after-meal reaction is even worse if they consume processed carbohydrates, which cause a state of hyperglycemia.

Glucose is the form in which carbohydrates are digested and absorbed. Immediately after a high-carbohydrate meal, an unnatural rise in blood glucose signals the body to pump lots of insulin into circulation to handle the excess glucose. The excess insulin lowers the blood glucose so severely that a state of hypoglycemia results.

The up-and-down glucose absorption in these children is exacerbated by their other metabolic problems. The hyperglycemic phase causes hyperactivity and self-stimulation in autistic kids, and the hypoglycemic phase causes headaches, tantrums, fatigue, and more. All the child knows is that she doesn't feel well.

The solution is to emphasize unprocessed, high-fiber, low-starch fruits, vegetables, and grains, which get absorbed more slowly, resulting in a gradual increase in blood glucose. This is the way the human body was designed to handle carbohydrates. If each meal includes high-protein and high-fiber foods, along with adequate fat to slow down digestion, everyone will be happier.

> ### DEFINITIONS
>
> - Hyperglycemia: High blood sugar. Symptoms include hyperactivity and self-stimulation in spectrum children.
>
> - Hypoglycemia: Low blood sugar. Symptoms include disorientation, headache, verbal difficulty, shakiness, anxiety (and tantrums in children), and fatigue.

If breakfast consists of processed, sugary cereal…well, you can predict that the rest of the day will be downhill. You can expect another day filled with behavioral abnormalities at school, where the only thing your child learns seems to be aggression and new ways to be distracted.

To prevent or relieve hypoglycemic episodes, eliminate candy and sugary fruits or fruit juices, and every hour or two eat some protein or low-starch vegetable. To keep the spikes and swings to a minimum, at mealtime and snack time emphasize low-sugar, high-fiber fruits; no fruit juice; low-starch vegetables (very limited high-starch, low-fiber vegetables such as corn and potatoes); poultry; lean meats; fish; eggs; limited servings of whole sprouted grains; and avoid all sweets.

Processed carbohydrates are essentially "toxic" to the child's system, and they have a detrimental effect on the beneficial gut flora while they feed pathogenic bacteria and funguses that are causing the dysbiosis and food allergies. Processed carbs also weaken the immune system and undermine resistance to infections.

If your child has been on the GF/CF diet for one to three months and has the symptoms of hypoglycemia, you should get his blood glucose level checked as soon as possible and make dietary modifications as recommended.

THE SPECIFIC CARBOHYDRATE DIET (SCD)

The percentage of spectrum children who require modifications of the GF/CF diet continues to increase. Why? Because even on a GF/CF diet (and even if that diet has been augmented by an anti-hypoglycemic diet and/or an anti-yeast diet), unwelcome gut bacteria and yeast can continue to flourish, feeding on the carbohydrates that are not fully digested due to enzyme deficiencies. Specifically, the culprit is disaccharides. Carbohydrates need to be eliminated, so that the bacteria will die off. You need to limit sugars to monosaccharides (fructose and glucose), the simple sugars found in non-starchy fruits and vegetables, which are well-tolerated by 4-A kids. This is the specific carbohydrate diet (SCD).

How can you tell if you should consider the SCD for the sake of your child's healing? Assuming you have given the current diets a fair and lengthy trial, does your son or daughter still suffer from gastrointestinal symptoms such as abdominal pain, diarrhea with intermittent constipation, gas, and bloating? In addition does your child continue to have the same cognitive and behavioral issues?

If so you should consider undertaking the SCD. You will need to look for guidance because the diet is very specific, and it is important to stick closely to every guideline.[6]

Here is the general outline of the specific carbohydrate diet:

Not allowed

- Grains and flour (besides wheat and other gluten-containing grains, eliminate rice, corn, oats, rye, buckwheat, millet, quinoa, tapioca, and bulgur—this means no bread, no crackers, no chips, no pasta, and no popcorn)
- Starchy vegetables (such as potatoes or yams)
- Sugar and sweeteners except honey and saccharine
- Jams, jellies, or catsup
- Canned vegetables or fruits
- Dairy products, except perhaps homemade yogurt
- Soy or rice milk, canned coconut milk
- Soft drinks
- Processed meats (lunch meat, hot dogs, breaded meats or fish, or canned meat)
- Roasted nuts, glazed nuts, mixed nuts (often starch-coated)
- Processed fats (for example, margarine)

Allowed

- Meats and fish (fresh or frozen only, preferably organic and mercury-free)
- Meat and fish stock (homemade)
- Nuts (preferably purchased in shells, no additives)
- Seeds (such as sunflower, pumpkin, and sesame; preferably slightly sprouted for easier digestion and increased nutrient availability)
- Eggs (preferably organic from free-range hens)
- Vegetables (fresh or frozen only, preferably organically grown)
- Beans (pinto beans, soybeans, chick peas, and some others)
- Fruits (no sugar added, ripe [unripe fruit is starchy], preferably served separately from meat; do not serve if your child has diarrhea)

- Fruit juices (preferably made at home, no additives, no pasteurization)
- Almond or coconut milk (homemade only)
- Honey (natural)
- Fats and oils (organic butter; cold-pressed olive, flaxseed, and avocado oils; natural meat fats)

Naturally, you will need to factor in the special needs of your child. Does he balk at eating foods of certain textures? This problem, so typical of spectrum children, may disappear of its own accord as healing progresses, but there is no use forcing her to choke down foods that repel him. Is he genuinely allergic to some foods? Omit those foods from her diet, even if they are on the "allowable" list.

> You will need to factor in the special needs of your child.

Because the diet is so strict, you may need to start slowly with easy-to-digest foods. Many ordinary foods that are allowable on the SCD, such as peanuts and beans, are nevertheless difficult for a child with a compromised gastrointestinal system to digest. Wait until the gut heals before you introduce the harder-to-digest foods on the SCD list.

For a detailed list of allowable and forbidden foods on the SCD you can refer to the list on the website www.pecanbread.com[7] as well as other sources. The SCD has been around for more than sixty years, helping people with all sorts of digestive disorders, including celiac disease, Crohn's disease, and ulcerative colitis.

You should know ahead of time that when your child starts the SCD, he or she may feel ill. This is because the unwelcome bacteria are dying off en masse, creating die-off toxins and accompanying symptoms. This may make compliance with the new diet more difficult than ever. However, if you persevere (perhaps keeping allowable snacks on hand that your child enjoys), you will be rewarded with a healthier child. Warm Epsom salt baths may help. Go slow on probiotics and yogurt. You can head off these symptoms to some degree if you gradually decrease the amount of sugar and starches in your child's diet for at least a week before launching the SCD.

You will know that the diet is working when these symptoms subside, along with other "normal" (to your child) symptoms of inflammation and dysbiosis. If it works, it's certainly worth the trouble. As Dr. Sidney Baker, cofounder of Defeat Autism Now! (DAN!), wrote in the book *Autism: Effective Biomedical Treatments,* "SCD is the best treatment that I have found so far for many children on the autism spectrum."[8] If your child's symptoms do not subside, feel free to discontinue the diet.

As it turns out, as stringent as it may be, an SCD is an excellent method for becoming optimally nourished, whether or not a person has one of the 4-A disorders. I mention that only because you may discover that your entire family might be able to use the same diet, thus simplifying food preparation. I am recommending the SCD as a first choice for 4-A kids. I also start them on betaine hydrochloride with pepsin for their low stomach acid.

ISSUES SURROUNDING SOY

Some 4-A kids will need to be on a gluten-free, casein-free, soy-free (GF/CF/SF) diet. Why is this? Isn't soy supposed to be good for you?

Soy products are very inexpensive to produce, and the food market exploded with them following research that showed soy had health-promoting benefits. Although the health benefits were found in studies on people who consumed fermented soy in their diets (tofu, miso, tempeh), the soy that ends up in many foods is in the form of soy protein isolate, which is processed soy containing aluminum and nitrates, both of which have been implicated in nervous system disorders. Soy infant formulas contain this product. Also, soy can interfere with the absorption of iodine in the thyroid gland, which can contribute to hypothyroidism, which can have far-ranging effects on growth and development, including brain maturation. Our 4-A kids are notoriously deficient in calcium, magnesium, iron, and zinc, but the phytates in soy bind those minerals, reducing absorption and further depleting these mineral stores. Extensive allergy testing for soy in autistic children has found many of them to be allergic to it. The phytoestrogens in soy fed to infants and young children can lead to endocrine hormone problems.

However, fermented soy products may be considered beneficial for 4-A kids unless Candida overgrowth prevails and severe allergies to fermented foods has developed.

In general I recommend avoiding soy in 4-A diet plans.

LOW OXALATE DIET

As mentioned in chapter 4, oxalate is a highly reactive molecule that is abundant in many plant foods. But when it is present in human cells in high amounts, it can lead to oxidative damage, depletion of glutathione, the igniting of the immune system's inflammatory cascade, and the formation of injurious crystals that are accompanied by pain. Ordinarily not much oxalate is absorbed from the diet, but the level of absorption has to do with the condition of the gut. When the gut is inflamed or leaky and there is poor fat digestion, excess oxalate from foods can be absorbed from the GI tract and affect other cells in the body. A low oxalate diet may benefit 4-A kids, especially if other diets have failed to produce adequate results. The diet is designed to reduce or eliminate the oxalate that the child consumes in food.

> **ACRONYMS FOR TYPES OF DIETS**
> - GF/CF: gluten-free/casein-free diet
> - GF/CF/SF: gluten-free/casein-free/soy-free diet
> - SCD: specific carbohydrate diet

Does your child complain of a tummy ache within a couple hours of eating a meal? Are fatty foods a particular problem? Is your child always running to the bathroom to urinate (and perhaps bed-wetting at night)? Has chronic constipation or diarrhea been a pattern? Most tellingly, does your child crave foods that are high in oxalate? (See list below.)

Benefits reported by parents using the low oxalate diet, according to researcher Susan Owens, include the following:

- Improvements in gross and fine motor skills
- Improvements in expressive speech
- Better counting ability
- Better receptive and expressive language
- Increased imitation skills
- Increased sociability
- Speaking in longer sentences
- Decreased rigidity
- Better sleep
- Increased imaginary play
- Improved cognition
- Loss of bed-wetting
- Loss of frequent urination
- Improved handwriting
- Improved fine motor skills
- Improvement in anemia
- …and many more[9]

HIGH OXALATE FOOD LIST

Below is a representative list of foods that are high in oxalate (more than 7 milligrams of oxalate per serving). Foods marked with an asterisk have extremely high amounts of oxalates and should be completely eliminated.[10]

- Almonds
- Beans, green
- Beans (baked, dried, kidney)
- Beets (tops, roots, greens)
- Blackberries
- Blueberries
- Cashews
- Celery
- Chives

- Chocolate*
- Chocolate milk
- Cinnamon
- Cocoa
- Collards
- Dandelion
- Eggplant
- Escarole
- Fig cookies
- Figs (dried)
- Fruitcake
- Ginger
- Graham crackers
- Grapes (purple)
- Green peppers
- Grits (white corn)
- Kale
- Kiwi fruit
- Leeks*
- Lemon peel*
- Lime peel*
- Marmalade
- Mustard greens
- Okra*
- Orange peel
- Parsley
- Parsnips
- Peanut butter*
- Peanuts*
- Pecans*
- Pepper (more than 1 tsp./day)*
- Pokeweed*
- Raspberries
- Red currants
- Rhubarb*
- Rutabagas
- Sesame seeds
- Sorrel
- Soybean crackers*
- Soy protein*
- Soy sauce
- Spinach*
- Strawberries
- Summer squash
- Sunflower seeds
- Sweet potatoes*
- Swiss chard*
- Tangerines
- Tofu (soybean curd)*
- Tomato soup
- Vegetable soup
- Walnuts
- Watercress
- Wheat germ*
- Yams

As with the other diets you will want to monitor your child's symptoms as you restrict the foods that contain oxalate. Your child may have periodic unhappy periods when physical and emotional symptoms flare up. This is normal, although it is difficult to endure. (You may decide to undertake extra detoxification measures to help; see chapter 11.) See Appendix E for a source for recipes that are not only low oxalate but also GF/CF and SCD.

The low oxalate diet is a difficult diet for both parent and child. But it will be worth all the hard work and unpleasantness if your child turns out to be one of the ones who benefit from it.

ARE WE THERE YET?

This information can be overwhelming. If you look at the lists of forbidden foods and beverages for more than one of these diets at the same time, you begin to wonder if you can give your child anything at all to eat.

But everything can be taken in stages and steps, and you do not need to remember everything. Collect advice and lists from literature and websites such as the ones recommended in Appendix E. When you or your child slips up, which will happen inevitably, simply get back up and try again.

If, after you give the GF/CF diet a fair trial (being careful about yeast-promoting foods and allergic responses), your child seems to need more nutritional intervention, consider the SCD or the low oxalate diet. Find a knowledgeable nutritionist or integrative physician to help you along the way. Get on board with a supportive group of fellow parents who are trying the same things. None of these diets promise to solve all of your child's problems, but none of them will make them worse either, and they might just provide the breakthrough you've been looking for.

DIETARY INTERVENTION SUPPORT GROUPS

Help may be available from support groups in your area. Online, groups include the following:

- Gluten-Free/Casein-Free Diet (GF/CF): www.yahoogroups.com/group/gfcfkids

- The Specific Carbohydrate Diet (SCD): www.yahoogroups.com/group/pecanbread

- The Low Oxalate Diet: www.yahoogroups.com/group/Trying_Low_Oxalates

Chapter 10

✛ ?! 🐾 ❀

HEALING THROUGH
SUPPLEMENTATION THERAPY

Will had been diagnosed as a "spectrum child" about two years before his mother brought him in to see me when he was four years old. Like all autistic children Will had numerous allergies, the symptoms of which manifested on his skin as eczema. Also since birth he had manifested a peculiar repetitive movement of his head; his neck muscles would flex his head, which turned down and to the right side. This occurred many times a day and appeared to be a motor tic.

Will's mom was having a very difficult time changing her son's eating habits, so nutritional therapies had been minimally effective. Will's communication, cognitive, and behavior problems were severely limiting his progress. Nevertheless I formulated a plan based on updated laboratory studies and a new dietary program (SCD). But before we started, I told Will's mom that I wanted Will to begin taking a particular whole-food concentrate supplement. (See Appendix D.) I explained that the supplement would furnish Will with thousands of vitamins, minerals, and enzymes that he could never eat enough food on a daily basis to obtain, even if he had been compliant. This was the only therapeutic recommendation I made to begin with.

Within two weeks she called me, and I could tell she was crying as she tried to speak. "Dr. C., I'm looking at a miracle—Will's motor tic is gone!" In the course of the next month Will began to crave the fruits and vegetables from which the concentrate was derived. Soon thereafter he began to show improvements in all areas; definitive progress was evident. To me this proved to be a landmark proof of the value of supplementation with 4-A children.

SUPPLEMENTS—NOT OPTIONAL

You, like many people, may presume that you and your child should be able to get plenty of nutrients because of our abundant American diet. After all, isn't our main problem overeating? But the standard American diet is calorie and energy dense but nutrient poor.

Though we all need supplements, 4-A children have elevated needs. They do not fit the "minimum daily requirements" percentages. Without supplementation they are never going to achieve nutritional health.

Supplements—from vitamins and minerals to amino acids, enzymes, essential fatty acids, and other substances (sometimes derived from exotic-sounding sources)—are simply not optional for 4-A children. They need them to make up for their many deficiencies. Some of them need supplements to help them eliminate substances that their bodies produce too much of. (For instance, autistic kids tend to have too much copper and glutamate in their bodies, and it's not good for their nervous systems.) These kids need supplements to facilitate metabolic healing. And they need them to supply components of their basic nutrition in a consistent, controlled manner.

As I have mentioned earlier, 4-A kids are often picky eaters. As a result, they will eat only a narrow range of foods, and those foods are often nutrient-poor. In addition 4-A kids often suffer from abnormal enzyme function, which results in inadequate digestion. The mucosal lining of their guts are often inflamed, and food absorption can be very poor. Many of them suffer from abnormal bowel motility, coping with diarrhea or constipation or both on a regular basis. Even if they take supplements, the nutrients pass right through their systems without being absorbed. Topping that off is the simple fact that our American food supply is more nutrient-poor than it used to be, due to large-scale agricultural operations, long-distance shipping, and manufacturing/processing practices (think of "enriched bread").

COMMON NUTRIENT DEFICIENCIES AND DEPENDENCIES IN AUTISTIC CHILDREN[1]

- Calcium
- Selenium
- Zinc
- Magnesium
- Iron
- Cysteine
- Sulfate
- Taurine

- Vitamin B_{12}
- Vitamin B_6
- Lysine
- Methionine
- Essential fatty acids
- Vitamin D
- Vitamin E
- Vitamin A

Besides the deficiencies that come with the territory for a 4-A child, they also must cope with an increased need for nutrients because of varying amounts of exposure to environmental chemicals and pollutants.

WHICH SUPPLEMENTS ARE BEST?

There is no single, specific set of supplements for all 4-A children. The supplementation program must be individualized for the needs of each child. I take a careful look at the particulars of what the child needs—and doesn't need. What does he need more of? What does the child need to get rid of? How is the child responding to our efforts so far? I consider myself half of the physician-parent team. Together we must work closely to monitor progress and make appropriate adjustments along the way.

Before supplementation is begun, a thorough nutritional analysis should be performed. What does the child presently eat and drink? What are the child's cravings? What does the child refuse to try? Further, what foods seem to create problems for the child? What kinds of problems occur? Does the child have chronic gas, diarrhea, or constipation? What clues to unmet nutritional needs come from the child's hair, fingernails, or skin? The child's gums and eyes? Her demeanor?

We determine where to start by taking a long look at the child's digestive function. Given his current allergies, intestinal dysbiosis or leaky gut, age, abilities, and more, I add as many laboratory tests as necessary to ascertain what is being absorbed.

> Supplements—from vitamins and minerals to amino acids,
> enzymes, essential fatty acids and other substances—
> are simply not optional for 4-A children.

I make the selection of supplements myself, keeping in mind not only efficacy but also cost and likelihood of compliance. After all, what good is it to force the parents to abandon the regimen midstream because it costs too much or because their child refuses or finds it impossible to swallow so many pills? (Regarding pill-swallowing, you can look for supplements that come in small sizes or in a kid-friendly chewable or liquid form, if that doesn't introduce problematic dyes or flavors. Or you can pulverize tablets yourself and mix them with an easy-to-eat food that your child will tolerate.)

With any supplement, always start on the low side. If no change is seen at first, increase the dosage within known limits. If adverse effects ensue, simply discontinue the supplement. Bear in mind that supplements of digestive enzymes and probiotics may cause an initial adverse reaction, followed by a strong positive effect. The rule is to proceed with caution.

Wherever possible introduce supplements one at a time, so that you can tell which ones are working or creating problems. Keep complete and accurate records; it will be hard to remember the details otherwise. Especially with children with known allergies, remember to scrutinize the composition of supplements for potential problem substances. It won't serve anybody's purposes if you start a supplementation program that introduces an allergen into the mix.

In order to "supplement smart," you will need some sources of reliable information, even if your doctor is a specialist in this regard. For detailed information about nutritional supplements that has been compiled with 4-A children in mind, I recommend two books in particular: *Autism: Effective Biomedical Treatments* by Jon Pangborn, PhD, and Sidney M. Baker, MD; and *Healing the New Childhood Epidemics* by Kenneth Bock, MD, especially the supplement information on pages 257 292.

SOME ALTERNATIVE THERAPIES

Not all supplements are nutritional. Some are alternative therapies that may enhance the recovery of your child's highly unique needs. Below I explore several that may be of interest to you.

Melatonin therapy for sleep disorders

Melatonin (N-acetyl-5-ethoxytryptamine), a hormonelike molecule, is produced and elaborated from the pineal gland, but most tissues can produce it. Light inhibits it, so it begins to circulate in our bodies in the evening, which of course helps prepare us for the night's sleep. This hormone has an extremely important role in many functional systems. It regulates sleep, aids in brain development, and serves as a strong detoxifier and antioxidant. Research has shown that sleep is needed for metabolic restoration of the brain and for cognitive development. Healthy sleep is necessary to prevent disturbed behavior and cognitive and memory difficulties.

A majority of spectrum children experience sleep disturbances, and the problem can last for years. In my thirty years of pediatric practice I have noticed an increasing percentage of "normal" children (infants to teens) with sleep problems—at the present time about 80 percent of my patient population. Children have problems falling asleep, frequent awakenings during the night, and early-morning awakenings. Interestingly the rate of increase appears to be keeping pace with that of the 4-A epidemic. Perhaps this is not so surprising, since all of us have been exposed to the environmental causes of the 4-A epidemic.

Melatonin supplementation can help. It is readily available in controlled-release tablets that provide either fast-acting melatonin (to promote sleep for three or four hours at the beginning of the night) and slow-release melatonin (to promote sleep for an entire night of six to eight hours). These supplements can treat both sleep onset and sleep maintenance difficulties.

Children with ADHD may understand that it is time for them to sleep, but their over-excited brain circuits do not give the required signals to initiate pineal melatonin secretion until too late; as a result they have a chronic problem with delayed sleep onset. Oral melatonin bypasses their delayed signaling and promotes sleep within thirty minutes.

Circadian rhythm sleep disturbances (difficulty falling asleep, frequent awakenings, and early-morning awakenings) are characteristic for spectrum (autistic/ADD) children. Several studies have shown that melatonin therapy has a high success rate for combating delayed sleep onset and for providing longer sleep maintenance. Parents report that these same children improved in their health, behavior, and learning ability. Since

DEFINITIONS

- Motor tic: A repeated twitching of a group of muscles, either simple such as eye-blinking or complex such as twirling in place. Vocal tics involve the muscles that produce speech. Tics arise from the part of the brain that controls automatic movements and impulsivity.

- Glutamate: An amino acid (a building block for proteins) and a neurotransmitter in the central nervous system.

- Melatonin: A hormone that helps control the sleep cycle as well as other functions.

- Analgesic: Pain reliever.

- Vasoactive: Causing dilation or constriction of the blood vessels.

melatonin has antianxiety properties, it comes as no surprise that parents also report a reduction in anxiety and self-stimulating behavior. In fact, melatonin can be given during the day before medical procedures such as MRIs and EEGs because it calms children and helps them be more cooperative.

> Not all supplements are nutritional. Some are alternative therapies that may enhance the recovery of your child's highly unique needs.

How can you tell if you should try melatonin therapy? First determine if healthy sleep habits have been established, but sleep disturbances persist. You might decide to initiate therapy after only a two-week review of the child's sleep patterns (going to bed, falling asleep, awakenings, and associated behaviors).

Dr. James Jay, a pioneer in melatonin therapy for the sleep disorders of spectrum children, writes:

> In our experience, when children are tired and sleepy, they are usually ready to go to bed and fall asleep. It is when they cannot fall asleep that they may exhibit difficult bedtime behaviors. In such situations it may be wiser to treat them with melatonin first to correct their medical deficiency, and then the difficult behaviors might diminish or disappear. Certainly behavioral therapies are more successful when the children are not exhausted.[2]

Aromatherapy

Aromatherapy is the practice of using essential plant-derived oils to bring health to a person's body and mind. I believe that the fragrances and other qualities of the specially prepared, concentrated oils have untapped value in the treatment of 4-A children, and that aromatherapy may be able to uniquely address the underlying emotional needs of children who cannot express themselves well.

Essential oils have mood-altering properties. The sense of smell operates differently from the senses of sight, hearing, touch, and taste, which connect directly to the cerebral cortex, where a person thinks and reasons objectively and unemotionally. These four senses do not directly stimulate one's emotions. The sense of smell passes signals first to the emotional portion of the brain and stimulates the rational brain second.

When a 4-A condition has been partially derived from buried emotions, essential oils can release the impediments to healing. Children are observably relieved from their stresses and experience peace and calmness. Like adults in research studies, they may also experience improved cognitive function.[3] Studies of human olfaction (smell) have potential application for the treatment of 4-A children in the future. For example, several recent studies have shown that intermittent exposure to the fragrances of essential oils can help subjects sustain attention more efficiently. Proponents of aromatherapy claim that the benefits of essential oils include emotional, physical, and spiritual well-being; detoxification; antimicrobial action; antioxidant action; air purification; and stimulated circulation (which increases oxygen and nutrient delivery).

When an autistic, nonverbal adolescent smells fresh-cut grass, the scent triggers memories in the nonverbal portion of his brain that stores feelings and emotions, and he can remember a summer spent as a child on his grandfather's farm. Memories of emotions need some trigger for retrieval. Once such memories have been retrieved, the child can deal with them in a manageable way. I suspect that a spectrum child must possess an inordinate amount of repressed emotional trauma. Being noncommunicative, the child's opportunities to deal with the emotions and effect-increased healing through the normal means are severely restricted.

As always each child is different. To further pursue this alternative therapy and to tailor its application to your 4-A child, you will have to experiment. By and large children will not have a negative reaction to essential oils, although you may need to be careful of allergic reactions to some substances or derivations.

Inflammation-reducing supplement

To reduce gut and brain inflammation in the autistic-ADD population, I recommend a supplement called NeuroProtek.[4] A nutraceutical (dye- and preservative-free), it is formulated with flavonoids from green plants and seeds, unrefined olive kernel oil, and chondroitin sulfate.

Flavonoids reduce oxidative stress and inflammation, but they are not consumed in adequate quantities in most diets, and they are poorly absorbed; olive oil enhances absorption and chondroitin sulfate helps protect gut wall integrity.

The rationale of the formulators of this supplement is that autism is the result of a breakdown of the gut/blood and blood/brain barrier functions, which allows neurotoxic molecules to cause brain inflammation and faulty nerve processing. The immune cells known as mast cells can cause immune-mediated allergic reactions when they are activated by environmental, infectious, or allergic triggers, and stress, especially during gestation and immediately after birth. So if mast cell activation leads to gut, blood, and brain barrier disruption, permitting neurotoxic substances to enter the brain, autism may be the result.

The majority of spectrum children have a family history of allergies, and autistic symptoms worsen when the autistic child's allergies flare up. Since mast cells are located near blood vessels of the gut and brain, gut and brain permeability is increased when the mast cell neuron reactions occur. The triggers for these mast cell activations are environmental toxins and infectious agents (bacterial or viral). Once the mast cells are activated, they secrete vasoactive, neurosensitizing , and proinflammatory substances.

Flavonoids inhibit the release of proinflammatory substances and inhibit mast cell activation. NeuroProtek appears to take down the inflammation; initial trials with this product have shown promising results, and parents have reported significant improvements in communication skills and social interactions, especially after a period of months. Like other supplements it is not a definitive cure, and it should be used under the supervision of an informed doctor.

In conclusion remember that no supplement should be considered a cure for the 4-A disorders. Though you may see improvement in your child's health, even drastic improvement as with little Will at the beginning of this chapter, what you have accomplished is to shore up the overall physical and mental health of your child. This is an essential achievement, and it strongly undergirds all your other efforts. As your child's recovery takes hold, you will be able to discontinue some supplements or move on to new ones.

Chapter 11

HEALING THROUGH DETOXIFICATION THERAPY

Little Jill, who was nine years old, had dysfunctional sensory integration, which made her an especially poor eater. The sight, smell, and taste of food could cause her to become nauseated. She had severe asthma and sensitivities. The few foods she did eat all too frequently would become the source of severe inflammatory gut reactions, allergic in nature, that eventually caused "leaky gut," which allowed toxins to enter her bloodstream and find their way to her lungs, causing asthma attacks. Jill's doctor-parent team, realizing that nutrition and supplements were not proving to be effective in controlling her asthma, decided to step up her power to detoxify. She began daily Epsom salt baths, spent more time in hot saunas, and began to use infrared saunas. Her mother made her smoothies with food, herbs, and spices that enhanced her body's ability to synthesize glutathione. For months she massaged glutathione gel into Jill's skin every third day. She also increased her consumption of water. Vigorous exercise to promote sweating and rebounding became part of her normal routine. Within two months Jill began to enjoy more and more asthma-free days in a row.

A boy named Daniel is a high-functioning autistic seven-year-old with ADHD. When he was diagnosed at age two and a half, he had suffered from the classic signs and dysfunctional symptoms of his digestive system, his immune system, and his nervous system. His symptoms had improved with the correction of dysbiosis, the elimination of food allergies through a gluten- and casein-free diet, and supplementation with whole-food concentrate (see Appendix D), essential fatty acid, and other supplements to correct various deficiencies. However, when he turned seven, he suffered a relapse of symptoms. As it turned out, he had received numerous silver-mercury amalgam fillings in the intervening years, and a new review of his current dietary preferences showed a craving for tuna fish. With removal of his fillings and dietary modifications, he experienced a dramatic change in his health and improvements in all his symptoms. His cognitive and behavioral problems improved significantly. Chelation with dimercaptosuccinic acid (DMSA) also helped. Laboratory studies showed high levels of mercury in his urine.

"TOXED-OUT" KIDS

As you know, many complex factors have contributed to the 4-A epidemics. However, in the opinion of most integrative medical professionals who treat these children, many of these factors could be conquered or at least better tolerated if only the child's natural detoxification system could keep up with immune dysfunction, gastrointestinal dysbiosis, insufficient nutrition, and microbial invasion. It cannot.

In fact, toxins, in particular heavy metals such as mercury, as well as chemical environmental toxins may be to blame in the first place for the disordered body functions of 4-A children.

The only solution is to aggressively go after the polluting substances that have played havoc with these children's bodies. This counterattack is called detoxification. The goal of detoxification is threefold: (1) to reduce toxic buildup in the body cells; (2) to reduce inflammation in the gastrointestinal system, the immune system, and the nervous system; and (3) to reduce oxidative stress throughout the child's body.

In the chemistry of a healthy body, detoxification removes the chemical substances that are no longer needed or wanted. The detoxification treatments described in this chapter are designed to enhance and supplement the body's natural detoxification process.

When the body must remove a toxic molecule, it must synthesize another molecule to attach it to and make it less toxic. The combined molecules exit the body as waste products through urination, defecation, perspiration, and the growth and shedding of the hair and nails. This detoxification process is most active at night. Thus, if it is somewhat dysfunctional, sleep problems can result.

Glutathione, a powerful antioxidant that is often low in 4-A children, must be furnished by supplementation. Supplementary magnesium, niacin, and vitamin B_6 have also been shown to improve detox chemistry.

> The goal of detoxification is threefold: (1) to reduce toxic buildup in the body cells; (2) to reduce inflammation in the gastrointestinal system, the immune system, and the nervous system; and (3) to reduce oxidative stress throughout the child's body.

With sick 4-A children, I test the success of detoxification with "probes." I give the child caffeine or acetaminophen (Tylenol) by mouth or injection, and then retrieve them in the blood or urine to analyze them for changes. We're looking to see if the detoxification process took place. If these substances were not captured and ushered out of the body, we know we need to intensify our fight against toxins.

Where does the child's body pick up these toxins? Just about everywhere in our environment. It's hard to avoid exposure to pesticides and herbicides, solvents, formaldehyde, air and water pollution, and much more. Our food supply, our homes and schools, our automobiles—all contribute to the load. Bodily havoc can be caused by food additives alone—dyes, preservatives, MSG, artificial sweeteners, hormones, antibiotics, and more. Sometimes the very medicines that are meant to help us contribute toxins instead.

Then we have our own internal toxic generators in the form of metabolic waste, by-products of bacterial action, and dead matter in our GI tracts. Do you recall that strong urine smell in a neglected public restroom? That's ammonia, and it's a natural by-product. All human metabolism creates waste products, but the bodies of 4-A kids have a compromised disposal and cleansing system, so the waste products build up and do damage. If you add the bacteria, funguses, viruses, and parasites that are present in normal life, but your body cannot adequately and efficiently fight them off and discharge the aftereffects, then you have additional toxicity.

GETTING CLEANED UP

The sine qua non for detoxification is nutrition. Everything starts in the gut where toxins (or toxicity) can give rise to a multitude of problems. My approach to healing through detoxification begins with optimizing gut (digestive) function, because it serves as a prerequisite to protect the vitality of our essential cells that make up the immune and nervous systems.

In brief here is my approach:

1. First I treat dysbiosis—the way the gut gets taken over by opportunistic (pathogenic) flora.

2. Next I identify and eliminate food allergens. I have learned that all kids—4-A or not—have food allergies.

3. Then I address casein/gluten sensitivities.

4. This is followed closely by identifying and removing toxic heavy metals from the child's system.

5. After that I administer supplementation with whole-food concentrates (see Appendix D) and essential fatty acids.

6. Finally we settle into the implementation of an ideal dietary plan to maintain a healthy balance within the child's body.

If symptoms caused by dysbiosis persist after the initial dietary and supplement therapy has begun, this usually means that the beneficial bacteria have been killed by antibiotics and yeast overgrowth has set in. Fungal organic acids can be found in the urine of children with persistent dysbiosis. To treat this, we begin a yeast- and mold-free diet and antifungal medicine. (Along the way, with any plan to achieve digestive health, an adequate intake of dietary fiber must be established. A fiber supplement such as flaxseed, psyllium seed, and food-grade cellulose may be an extremely helpful component in the child's diet.)

A low-carbohydrate, high-fiber diet provides the environment to promote the colonization of the gut with beneficial bacteria, especially when probiotic supplements are included in the plan. I also recommend lots of leafy vegetables, cruciferous vegetables (for example, broccoli, cauliflower, and cabbage), root vegetables (such as beets and carrots), and beans; and very limited grains and tubers, since they are starchy (includes potatoes, sweet potatoes, and yams). I recommend limiting fruit intake, because fruit is sweet, and of course I recommend limiting sugar itself.

Clean: The Revolutionary Program to Restore the Body's Natural Ability to Heal Itself, a book written by Alejandro Junger, MD, provides the most comprehensive detoxification program that I have studied thus far. The core concepts of the book are as follows:

1. Toxins and stress create obstacles for the normal functioning and self-healing capabilities of our bodies.

2. Modern eating habits and lifestyles pollute our bodies and don't provide the nutrients necessary for them to function at optimum levels.

3. By removing the obstacles and providing what is lacking, our bodies bounce back into health, energy is restored, and we begin to look and feel our best.[1]

Junger's Clean Program includes many elements besides a specialized diet and lots of water: exercise, massage, saunas, sleep, and activities that benefit the mind and soul. A chart called "Clean Program At-a-Glance" can be found on pages 189–190 of his book, or downloaded from his website.[2] Another resource I recommend is *Detoxification and Healing: The Key to Optimal Health,* by Sidney MacDonald Baker, MD.

CHELATION THERAPY FOR HEAVY METALS

Chelation therapy removes heavy metals (most commonly mercury, lead, and arsenic) from the body through the administration of chelating agents (frequently DMSA). A chelating agent makes chemical bonds with metal ions, resulting in a water-soluble complex that enters the bloodstream and gets excreted through normal body processes. It is best undertaken after gut dysbiosis is under control and overall good nutrition has been established.

Chelation is most commonly used in the treatment of autism and also sometimes in the treatment of ADHD, asthma, and allergies. Like every other therapy chelation is not a magic bullet, but in many children, it seems to be just what is needed.

Before recommending chelation, I make sure that my young patients need it by checking their lab results for heavy metal overload. After the lab tests but before the actual chelation procedure begins, I also prescribe an increase in supplemental minerals, because chelation can result in a deficit of helpful minerals that you are not trying to eliminate. Its other side effects can only be eliminated by not continuing with the chelation; they include increased hyperactivity, self-stimulating behaviors, and general irritability. For many parents and children, however, these side effects are less significant than the potential damage being done within the child's body by the heavy metal load.

> Chelation is not a magic bullet, but in many children,
> it seems to be just what is needed.

I always check ahead of time to make sure that we have taken care of the source of the heavy metals. We need to remove the sources of toxic exposure beforehand, or we will be back where we started before long. Does the child have mercury amalgam dental fillings? If so, it is possible that they are adding to the mercury load that the child has already been exposed to through environmental sources, mercury-based preservatives in vaccinations, or through food. If you can afford it, and if your child can handle that much time in a dentist's chair, a dentist can replace the fillings with composite fillings.

I also remind parents to avoid including mercury-tainted seafood in the family diet, including the ubiquitous canned tuna. Other large fish such as swordfish also contain high levels of mercury in their edible tissues. Other sources of heavy metal toxicity should also be considered, such as drinking water, foods that are not raised organically (or cooked in nonstick cookware), industrial emissions from coal-burning manufacturing plants, or lawn and garden products.

After also checking the child's kidney and liver function to make sure that it is up to the task of eliminating the mercury, we schedule the chelation procedure with a physician who has become expert in administering it. The chelating agent, most commonly in this case DMSA, can be administered orally, rectally (via suppository), or transdermally (via a skin ointment or cream). Therapy will proceed over a period of months in an on-and-off cycle, with periodic testing to determine progress. When only a trace of heavy metal is being excreted, the chelation period is complete.

CHEMICAL POLLUTION

The heavy chemical pollution to which all of us are subjected takes a great toll on 4-A children because of their compromised natural detoxification systems. Lab tests of blood or urine can help determine the levels of chemicals in your child's body. For example, to check for excessive formaldehyde exposure (from the child's home or schoolroom environment), the test measures the formic-acid level. If a particular commercial product or location cannot be avoided in order to reduce the child's exposure to the chemical—or if a reduced exposure makes little difference because the child's natural detoxification processes are faulty, you will know that the unwanted chemical is being stored in the fatty tissues of the child's body and that more aggressive measures are called for.

> **DEFINITIONS**
>
> - Chelation therapy: Chelation therapy removes heavy metals (most commonly mercury, lead, and arsenic) from the body through the administration of chelating agents (frequently dimercaptosuccinic acid, or DMSA). A chelating agent makes chemical bonds with metal ions, resulting in a water-soluble complex that enters the bloodstream and gets excreted through normal processes.
> - DMSA (dimercaptosuccinic acid): One of several chelating agents that make chemical bonds with metal ions, resulting in a water-soluble complex that enters the bloodstream and gets excreted through normal body processes.

To eliminate the excess nonfood-related chemicals that have been stored in the child's body and brain, a formal detoxification program must be initiated under the supervision of a doctor. As with other toxins you want to promote the elimination of the unwanted chemicals through the child's urine, bowel movements, perspiration, expired air, and saliva. Cold-pressed polyunsaturated oils, along with particular vitamins and nutrients, will help the child's liver bind the chemicals so that they can be excreted via the intestines in bowel movements. Vitamin B_3 can assist the process of mobilizing the chemical that has been stored in fat so that it can pass into the blood-stream. Physical exercise will speed up the blood flow throughout body tissues so that the unwanted chemicals, once released, can move more quickly to the skin to be expelled in the sweat or to the intestines or bladder to be excreted. Increased perspiration can also be achieved by the careful use of saunas, and massages can generally stimulate the child's circulation and mobilize body fat. Besides utilizing as many detox techniques as you can and learning which nutrients will help alter the chemicals and excrete them, always be sure to encourage your child to drink lots of purified water. Allergy specialist Doris Rapp, MD, puts it clearly:

> [Drinking a lot of liquid a day] will enhance the excretion of all types of waste products....Liquids help excrete body impurities and soften bowel movements. Urge your children to drink more water or fresh, pure, unsweetened, less-contaminated, organic fruit or vegetable juice between meals. You can create a nutritious soda pop by diluting pure organic fruit juice with a large amount of pure carbonated water. Many children drink only sweetened juices or soda pop, which may appeal more to their taste, but for many reasons these are not as beneficial for the body as pure, clean water.[3]

It's important to bear in mind that the extra excretion will also result in a loss of potassium and other salts, which must be supplied on a regular basis through supplements.

LIVING CLEAN

Obviously it is better to avoid exposure to toxic substances in the first place. You may need to modify not only your family diet but also your home environment. Your goal is to make it as easy as possible for your child's body to stay on top of toxicity (not to somehow hope to increase tolerance to toxic substances by repeated exposure). You can buy food that has been certified as organic—or even grow some of your own in an organic garden or containers. If you have old water pipes, you should make sure that they are not made of lead and are not soldered with lead. If they are, but you cannot move away, at least let the tap water run for a while when you first turn it on in the morning, because the water will have absorbed its highest lead content when it is not moving during the night.

If you live in a city with heavy air pollution and cannot move to a cleaner area, you can use a high-quality air-purifying machine in the room where your child spends the most time. Conversely, if the air outside is not as much of a problem as the air inside your home because of your heating system or furnishings or construction elements (that may be outgassing formaldehyde or another pollutant), make sure you can open your windows to air out the place, especially in the child's bedroom.

Look for information specific to your situation about how to avoid toxins in your food supply and environment. Your most up-to-date information will often come from selected websites, and I have provided a representative list of them at the end of this book in Appendix E, "For More Information."

Chapter 12

HEALING THROUGH MEDICATION

Claudia, a seventeen-year-old high school senior, complained of trouble concentrating, distractibility and disorganization, low energy, difficulty reading, and feelings of being overwhelmed by life. She had frequent panic attacks over simple daily tasks.

She was afraid of medication and wanted to deal with her problems in a natural way, using diets, exercise, and meditation. But unfortunately these efforts had little effect. As she approached graduation and life beyond high school, she knew she needed help in order to "get it together."

After a small dose of Ritalin had had a significant positive effect on her symptoms, she had been diagnosed with ADHD, type 2 (inattentive). On Adderall she felt even better. "I feel like I have access to much more of my own brain," she told me. Quite simply, when she's on medication, she feels more focused and more organized, with more consistent energy and more brain power. As her grades improve and her life feels more ordered, she feels hopeful about her future as she leaves home and begins life as a young adult.

I have had other ADHD patients like Claudia, who had tried many natural therapies but who only managed to break free of the grip of their symptoms when they started taking a prescription medication. Their comments are rewarding to read:

"On medication, I experienced an increased awareness of the world around me."

"It's like being given sight after having been blind."

"For the first time I feel that I am in charge of my life."

"I'm no longer intimidated by others, as I used to be."

"I used to think I was stupid. It seemed like everyone else could do more things than I could. I'm starting to believe that there may be intelligent life in my body."

INTEGRATIVE MEDICINE INTEGRATES MEDICINE

A basic premise of holistic, integrative medicine is that the body can heal itself if conditions are ideal. We've come a long way in learning how to create environments conducive to healing 4-A children. As we have come to better understand the causes and mechanisms of the complex symptoms that make up the 4-A disorders, we have improved our ability to detoxify both the environment that these children live in as well as their bodily systems. Careful further attention to nutrition and supplementation has taught us how to repair the damage and eliminate causes. We are glad about the fact that we no longer aim to merely suppress symptoms with medication (medication that, of course, not only "puts chemicals in your body" but is also expensive and often hard to monitor).

But the fact is that much of the symptom complexes of severely ill 4-A children remains shrouded in mystery. The precise pathophysiology is poorly understood, even by the "experts," so our attempts to eliminate underlying causes are too often minimally effective, and our damage control is meager.

The fact remains that too often the symptoms themselves obstruct therapeutic efforts. In other words, before effective natural therapies can take hold, at least some of the troublesome symptoms must be suppressed with appropriately chosen medicines.

This statement raises alarms in people who have learned to be suspicious of all things pharmacological. Yet the truth is that neither medicine, nor the companies that supply it, nor the physicians who prescribe it are the enemy. The disease is. Therefore, if you can suppress some or many of the debilitating symptoms of autism, ADHD, asthma, or allergies, you can provide both life-saving help for the young patient and a survival mechanism for the entire family dynamic. You can "buy time" for natural solutions to work. Often you cannot even get to square one with, say, a complex dietary modification unless you have the fullest possible cooperation from a young patient who, on her own without medical help for symptom control, cannot comply with the simplest protocols, let alone comprehend the importance of long-term persistence.

> Before effective natural therapies can take hold, at least some of the troublesome symptoms must be suppressed with appropriately chosen medicines.

Many of the natural therapies that eventually change the course of a 4-A disorder can take months to achieve positive outcomes. These kids need support to stay focused and to maintain self-control amidst their cognitive and behavioral problems. Neurotransmitter imbalances cause insomnia, depression, and eating disorders that will persist until a livable balance can be achieved with medications. Chronic infections and self-perpetuating dysbiosis, so very prevalent in 4-A children, absolutely require antimicrobial medication. Sometimes these children need such medication for a very long time, until their systems recover full function and can take over.

Granted, physicians and parents need to anticipate and prepare for possible side effects of such powerful medications, and they need to pay attention to protecting the very functional systems of the child that have already been compromised. For example, it can be extremely challenging to correct the delicate and fastidious nature of beneficial gut microflora once chronic medication therapy has caused its own dysbiosis. Drug-caused dysfunctions can cause severe digestive and immune problems, which makes it imperative that physicians and parents balance the relative benefits of choosing a particular medical approach. Just think of the potential serious food allergy and sensitivity reactions, the dysregulated immunity reactions, the deranged metabolism and chronic bowel inflammation that both require medicines—and sometimes result from them.

Kids who are suffering and are sometimes acutely ill do need medications such as anti-inflammatories and antimicrobials (antibiotics, antivirals, and antifungals), but you don't want to throw them to the wolves. As with everything else in this complex stew of health problems, you need to keep trying, stay flexible, and aim for the best results with the fewest additional new rules and expenses.

Because spectrum disorders are neurobiological in nature, effective treatment can depend on biological intervention. At the same time other interventions must always be engaged, and eventually they could replace the need for medication. The integration of pharmaceutical medications with holistic healing modalities must be not only allowed but also encouraged if we expect to help 4-A children.

With systems correction the child's neuropsychiatric symptomatology will change for the better. The 4-A disorders may be occurring at epidemic proportions, but each sufferer is an individual whose body has distinct requirements and limitations. Medications must be chosen based on the unique individual needs of each particular 4-A child.

To be sure, some kids are overmedicated. Others have had to learn the hard way that antidepressants or other mood-altering drugs have only complicated their recovery. But rather than overreacting and blaming the drugs and the physicians who prescribed them, we need to move on to other strategies.

How can you spot potential side effects early enough? If possible you can try out new medications when your child is not in the midst of a crisis. Then any unwanted side effects will be more obvious to you. For example, you could try a new asthma drug when your child's airways are clear to make sure that it doesn't have too much of a sedating effect. You don't always have to wait until you are forced to use a new medicine.

Medications must be wisely integrated with other lifestyle-changing therapies (diet and environmental). That's why I say, "Integrative medicine integrates medicine." By themselves medicines are not magic bullets or panaceas. But given the seriousness of the 4-A epidemic, we simply cannot get along without them. Sometimes they are crucial to survival (think of the emergency medical intervention that saves the life of a child in the throes of an asthmatic attack). Generally speaking, medications are valuable adjuncts to holistic caregiving.

The aim of all holistic physicians is to achieve healing for their patients so that they will no longer require drugs. Of course this is not always possible. Sometimes, for instance, a child's severe allergy to mold or another household contaminant cannot be alleviated by means of moving to another home, because the family simply cannot do it. Sometimes parents must juggle too many family and job responsibilities to permit them to monitor a complicated dietary program. Often medicines are the only practical choice, given the circumstances.

> ### DEFINITIONS
>
> - Pathophysiology: The study of the abnormalities of body function that characterize particular diseases or syndromes.
> - Neuropsychiatric symptomatology: The cognitive and behavioral symptoms of a disorder that include both psychic and organic aspects.

MEDICATIONS FOR AUTISM

Most of the drugs that are typically used to treat children on the autism spectrum are psychoactive medications, and they fall into two categories: (1) anticonvulsants and (2) antidepressants and stimulants.

The majority of these medications were not developed with autism in mind. Only after they had come into use for other disorders did doctors begin to use them for their young autistic patients.

Increasingly physicians are also using medicines to target the comorbid conditions such as infections that so frequently cause problems for their autistic patients. ("Comorbid" sounds frightening, but it only means that two or more medical conditions have been diagnosed in the same person. Typically these medical conditions go hand in hand.)

> By themselves medicines are not magic bullets or panaceas. But given the seriousness of 4-A epidemic, we simply cannot get along without them.

As you might suspect, drug treatments for autism in and of themselves do not result in a cure; the symptoms suppressed by a particular medicine will return once the drug is stopped.

Anticonvulsants can help with more than seizures, which may or may not be a part of a particular diagnosis of autism. Typically they affect a neurotransmitter known as gamma-aminobutyric acid (GABA), which helps control mood as well as muscle action. This can provide huge relief for the families of children whose mood cycles otherwise cause havoc or whose anxiety and panic attacks are out of control, particularly for autistic kids who have bipolar features as well.

Antidepressants have frequently been used to treat autism, and antipsychotic drugs run a close second. Since we're talking about children here, though, dosages can be difficult to adjust, and side effects can be hard to anticipate. Still, many kids on the autism spectrum need help with their serotonin function, and that's what antidepressants are designed to do. (Serotonin is a neurotransmitter that helps a person feel contented.) Antipsychotic drugs require close monitoring, but their potential benefits are worth it with children who are out of control. Here again, the risk of side effects is outweighed by the larger risks of self-injury and aggressive behavior. Allow me to quote Dr.

Bock, who has more experience than most of us in treating autistic kids with antipsychotic drugs:

> Although the potential side effects of these drugs can be daunting, I have not yet encountered any appreciable degree of severe side effects from these drugs in my own practice. As a rule, I keep the doses as low as possible, and use the medications only to control severe symptomatology. The most common debilitating side effect of this class of drugs has been weight gain, generally related to carbohydrate metabolism. I generally attempt to mitigate this weight gain through a lower carbohydrate diet, and nutritional supplements that enhance insulin sensitivity.
>
> Many of these atypical antipsychotic drugs have been tested for use in autism, and some of them show moderately positive effects against autism-spectrum disorders. They help control aggression, hyperactivity, irritability, self-injury, and tantrums. In one study of Risperdal—which is the only drug that has been approved specifically for autism—87 percent of the children experienced at least some degree of improvement.[1]

Stimulant drugs such as Ritalin can be used for some autistic kids, especially those who show many features of ADHD. (This illustrates once again the connection between these two 4-A disorders.) I use them at times to help kids comply with rigorous dietary and activity regimens. Adderall (mentioned above in Claudia's ADHD story) is not usually one of the recommended stimulants to prescribe for autistic children, because it pushes their dopamine levels too high.

The other medications that can be used to treat autism do not fall into one category. They include secretin (which helps autistic kids with GI problems, diarrhea in particular), low-dose lithium, and several other drugs that help small segments of the autism-spectrum children. In addition, of course, we often need to use antimicrobial drugs (antibiotics, antivirals, and antifungals) and anti-inflammatory preparations.

MEDICATIONS FOR ATTENTION DEFICIT HYPERACTIVE DISORDER

Medications used to treat ADHD should achieve one or more of the following outcomes. They should: (1) decrease restlessness or high activity levels, (2) decrease irritability, (3) increase motivation, (4) decrease impulsiveness and increase thoughtfulness, (5) decrease distractibility, and/or (6) increase attention span and learning. It is essential to choose the appropriate medication for each type of ADHD; otherwise the medicine will not work.

Speaking in general terms, I use: (1) stimulants for type 1 and 2; (2) medications to enhance serotonin and dopamine for type 3; (3) anticonvulsants for type 4; (4) stimulating antidepressant medication for type 5; and (5) anticonvulsants and stimulant medication for type 6.

Not only do the different types of ADHD call for different medications, each child differs from the others as well. Integrating prescription medications into a holistic treatment program must be highly personalized. And it is a fact that some children absolutely require medicines long-term while others can use them for a crucial period of time and then be weaned off them. Parents should make sure that they don't just keep refilling the prescription on the assumption that this is

DEFINITIONS

- **Psychoactive:** Affecting a person's mind. The word is used mostly to refer to drugs.

- **Antidepressant:** One of a number of types of drugs that helps counteract depression by aiding and improving a person's concentration, appetite, sleep, and mood.

- **Anticonvulsant:** A drug that decreases abnormal electrical activity within the brain, thus cutting down on the frequency and severity of seizures for someone with a seizure disorder; sometimes prescribed for people with other disorders.

- **Antimicrobial:** An agent that attacks microscopic organisms such as bacteria, funguses, and viruses.

- **Neurotransmitter:** A chemical released from a nerve cell to transmit a message to another nerve, muscle, organ, or some other body tissue.

- **Dopamine:** A brain chemical (neurotransmitter) associated with feelings of pleasure as well as with movement, emotion, and motivation. Low dopamine levels are predictable with attention deficit disorder and autism.

the sum total of available treatment. They should also, in cases of long-term medicine usage, make sure that their child's metabolism gets monitored. Nobody wants to add unwanted side effects to a helpful medication, especially if there's a chance that the child is being overmedicated.

Ritalin (generic name: methylphenidate) is the oldest and best-known ADHD medication. Other stimulant drugs, by brand name, include Concerta, Metadate, and Daytrana (all methylphenidate); Adderall, Focalin, Dexedrine, Destrostat, and Vyvanse, as well as the nonstimulant drug Strattera.

I prefer to use the newer forms of methylphenidate most of the time. Its effects are similar to those of amphetamines, only milder, and it calms children with ADHD, helping them with mental tasks.

Comorbid disorders occur with somewhat less severity in ADHD children compared to children with autism. The prescriptive treatments for comorbid disorders are the same as they would be for other children. Many times ADHD and its associated ailments respond well to natural therapies that get to the root of the problem.

> ## DEFINITIONS
>
> - Stimulant: A drug that works by increasing dopamine levels in the brain. Dosages increase gradually (so as to avoid "hyper" behavior or addiction) until the desired therapeutic effect has been reached.
>
> - GABA: Gamma-aminobutyric acid, a neurotransmitter that helps the brain maintain muscle control and mood.
>
> - Serotonin: 5-hydroxytryptamine, a neurotransmitting hormone that transmits nerve signals between nerve cells, causes blood vessels to narrow, and affects a person's level of contentment.

MEDICATIONS FOR ASTHMA

Medication is clearly life-saving with acute asthma attacks or status asthmaticus (a serious condition in which asthma attacks follow quickly after one another without a gap). Asthma drugs do not cure the disease; they only keep the symptoms under control.

Medications for asthma are principally bronchodilators and

anti-inflammatories. Asthma medicines are available in a wide variety of forms, including sprays, tablets, capsules, and injectables.

To successfully treat an asthmatic child (or adult), it is important to prevent attacks if it all possible or to medicate the person as early as possible and as aggressively as necessary before the spasms in the airways become more severe. Most asthmatic kids need medicines for quick relief in crucial situations as well as for general inflammation control. As part of a preventative program you should be sure to eliminate from your environment as many substances as possible to which your child may be allergic or sensitive. If Junior's asthma is exacerbated by his allergic reaction to cat dander, then you will have to find a new home for Fluffy. If every cold bug aggravates his asthma, you will need to help him to build up his resistance as cold season approaches. Commonly, where allergic reactions trigger asthmatic symptoms, parents rely on decongestant medications to keep inflammation and congestion under control. (See the next section, Medications for Allergies.) Both theophylline asthma drugs and beta-adrenergic (beta-agonists) help the muscle spasms to calm down, and they take down the associated swelling and production of extra mucus. They can be breathed directly into the lungs to give instant relief from the symptoms of an asthma attack. As helpful as they can be, these drugs should not be allowed to be overused by children, who easily learn how to use inhalers, because overuse can make the asthma worse by causing new spasms.

Theophylline drugs both relax the airways and keep histamine from being released. Side effects can be a concern with theophylline medications. A possible alternative can be a cromolyn sodium spray that is used prophylactically (to keep asthma attacks away), and its side effects are less worrisome. When it is used every day, the child's airways become less reactive and therefore less likely to spasm. Corticosteroids, which also must be used daily, counteract inflammation.

As always where any medication is introduced into the mix, the physician-parent team must always develop and maintain a high index of suspicion and vigilance for adverse responses to such powerful medications. The well-being of the child is of the utmost importance.

MEDICATIONS FOR ALLERGIES

As with asthma, medication can be life-saving with serious allergic or anaphylactic reactions. It can also be used on a more regular basis to control allergy symptoms. Antihistamines, decongestants, steroid inhalants, systemic steroids, and nutraceuticals can all be used, depending on the circumstances.

If the cause of an allergy cannot be eliminated, antihistamines may be needed for years, in spite of the fact that many of them inhibit alertness and may compromise a child's performance in school or sports. If you must rely on antihistamines, try to choose a preparation that causes the fewest side effects.

It should be mentioned that some allergic children will be sensitive to the ingredients in the very medicines that are supposed to help them. Be careful about dyes and artificial flavors in children's medicines, as well as other ingredients such as artificial sweeteners, sugar, and corn (found in corn syrup sweeteners).

To relieve nose stuffiness and reduce the risk of related problems with the ears, you can use nose drops or sprays (judiciously). If you use them all the time, the delicate tissues in the nasal passages can swell, creating a vicious cycle. The same is true for Vaseline-like preparations that contact the skin inside the nose.

For skin inflammations you can use cortisone creams. As with other drugs cortisone and steroid drugs are meant only for relief in

DEFINITIONS

- Status asthmaticus: A serious condition in which asthma attacks follow quickly after one another without a gap.

- Theophylline: A type of bronchodilator drug that can help control mild asthma, especially at night.

- Beta-agonists (beta-adrenergic drugs): Bronchodilator drugs that, when inhaled into the lungs, relieve asthma symptoms by relaxing the muscles around the bronchial tubes and keeping them relaxed.

- Corticosteroids: Anti-inflammatory drugs taken daily for long-term prevention of asthma attacks.

critical situations. With children especially, you should never use them in large doses or over the long term.

Needless to say, no medicine can provide a permanent answer to allergies. This means that no medicine can alleviate one of the underlying factors in the 4-A epidemic. Even immunotherapy, which can be quite effective in desensitizing children and adults to allergens, cannot claim to cure the condition. In any case they are not drugs per se but rather preparations of the very substances to which a person is allergic, administered in ever-increasing doses, vaccination-style.

COVERING THE BASES

I saved the topic of medicines until late in the book, because I am so intent on helping 4-A children and their families to make more natural choices for treatment. Still, for such complex and insidious disorders, it's undeniably true that we need to add pharmaceuticals to nutraceuticals and sensible life choices.

Medications can work quickly, and they can help in certain long-term situations. They can help correct a wide variety of physical disorders that can harm the brain. They can quickly control extreme behavioral symptoms and certain physical problems, they can help solve certain long-term issues, and they can correct many of the diverse physical factors that feed into the 4-A disorders.

Medication therapy must be an individual program for each child. And since you need holistic care, and almost for sure you will need prescriptions and medical advice from a medical point of view, I want to reiterate my advice about finding an integrative physician with whom to work.

As an integrative pediatrician I integrate the entire family dynamic when I advise a parent of a 4-A child. To some extent I am treating the entire family, and the entire family affects the child's response to other therapies. Sometimes the most humane approach includes judicious use of pharmaceuticals, simply to keep the afflicted child from commandeering 100 percent of the family's attention and energy. Besides attaining the blessed relief from symptoms, we need to find a way to get some breathing room—and of course I'm not just talking about asthmatics—in order to employ holistic methods that will promote further healing of the underlying causes of autism, ADHD, asthma, and allergies.

Conclusion

EMPOWERING PARENTS

I have always been impressed to see how the lives of the family members of ASD children have been affected by them permanently. Their parents impress me most of all; they become much better people as they learn how to love and guide their afflicted child. Siblings at first will pray that God would make their brother or sister "normal," but eventually they realize and accept that autism will always be with their brother or sister and that their whole family will be normal in a different way. Many of them describe the gifts their autistic brother or sister has given them, such as the gift of patience to deal with others and the ability to love and accept people just as they are.

Young couples who have just found out that their baby is on the autism spectrum are advised to seek the advice of other parents who have raised an autistic child from birth to adulthood. These older parents counsel them that one of the most important things to remember is that their autistic child is not capable of being anyone else. He or she is unable to act in any other way than the way dictated by the damaged, malfunctioning brain. While they may see improvement, they should expect that their child will never gain complete control of abnormal behaviors and that the goal should be maximizing as many functions as possible, while loving their child every minute of every day.

The more the abnormal behaviors are understood and accepted, the more the family will benefit and develop gratitude for any progress made throughout the individual's lifetime. Somehow, acceptance itself lends itself to progress—and teamwork. Truly understanding friends who believe in them and who help them find their way are a large part of the picture. Ideally, one of those friends would be their child's pediatrician.

PARENTS RISING UP

As you begin to realize the catastrophic nature and enormity of this epidemic (which has become very personal to you because of your own child), you must be asking yourself, as I have countless times: Why? How has the suffering of our children made a difference in the world? The response from men and women of science has been impressive, and we continue to accumulate knowledge at a dizzying rate. But how can *my* experience count?

After many hours of study in preparation for the writing of this book, I experienced an epiphany. We, along with all of our 4-A kids, are in this together. The causes of the 4-A epidemic are in and around all of us. All of us have been exposed. Once the causes of the 4-A epidemic have been recognized and we have begun to understand how to achieve healing, we must take this knowledge and apply it to our lives, to all living plants and animals, to the planet itself. This is a work in progress, and each one of us must rise up to make a difference in our own personal sphere of influence.

Young parents who have been conditioned to think that professionals know best and who therefore tend to give them authority over their 4-A children must be taught to realize that they know their own children better than anyone else. They are the ones who live with them full-time in their real-life context, and they are the ones who have observed them far more deeply than any professional ever can.

Parents need to become more confident in this knowledge. Groups of parents can do wonders, armed with this confidence. For example, consider the group of parents who visited their local state representative. They requested and were granted legislation that founded a summer school for special education students.

Parents of ASD kids have a wealth of common sense. Developing a support system of other parents is both priceless and effective at transmitting some of what has been learned in the trenches to policy makers and influential professionals. This can help shift the balance in the right direction, across state and national lines.

> We, along with all of our 4-A kids, are in this together.

It must begin with a paradigm shift in thinking about medical care. We must bring holistic, integrative medicine into the mainstream. As defined in 2004 by the Consortium of Academic Health Centers for Integrative Medicine, integrative medicine is the practice of medicine that (1) reaffirms the importance of the relationship between practitioner and patient; (2) focuses on the whole person; (3) is informed by evidence; and (4) makes use of all appropriate therapeutic approaches, health care professionals, and disciplines to achieve optimal health and healing.[1]

In order for us to apply the knowledge that we have acquired from our study of the 4-A epidemic, and in order to promote our own (personal and corporate) well-being, we must learn about and embrace the holistic, integrative medicine model of care.

Integrative medicine gives major emphasis to the importance of *relationship* in healing. Regardless of which healing modality the integrative practitioner employs, from acupuncture to drugs, it is the connection between the practitioner and patients that helps define the practitioner as holistic. The integrative doctor strives to communicate and maintain a connection with the patient.

FOSTERING THE INTEGRATIVE DOCTOR-PATIENT RELATIONSHIP

We must grasp the importance of the doctor-patient relationship in order to make it a mutual partnership.

Dr. K. B. Thomas published a study of two hundred patients, all of whom had symptoms such as cough, sore throat, and abdominal pain but for whom no definitive diagnosis could be made initially. The patients were divided into two groups. Half of the group was given a "positive" consultation in the form of a firm diagnosis, and they were told they would get better in a few days. The other half was given "negative" consultation, and they were told that the doctor could not determine what was wrong. Some of them were offered a placebo treatment, and the rest were offered no treatment at all. After two weeks, when they were asked how they felt, a significantly greater percentage of those given a positive consultation reported feeling better. Whether or not patients received prescribed treatment made no difference. The outcomes could be predominately predicted based simply on the type of communication between the doctor and patient.[2]

This illustrates the power of the physician-patient relationships, and it points to the effectiveness of integrative therapies. The practice of integrative medicine helps empower parents physically, emotionally, physiologically, and mentally for the tasks that they face on a daily basis, which are formidable. Successful implementation of dietary programs, detoxification protocols, and supplement recommendations is extremely challenging. It is one thing to prescribe a treatment, but it's quite another to achieve compliance and successful completion of a therapeutic program.

Parents need help. They need ongoing education, training, and coaching to successfully treat and heal their children. They also need to develop a belief in the achievability of healing. Parents must be taught how to develop a conscious determination to improve the health and well-being of their 4-A child, along with an expectation of improvement in health and a meaningful, productive life. They need hope—the belief that a desired health goal can be achieved even if it is not a complete cure.

Connection is essential. In a way this is nothing new, although we may have lost track of it. Healing modalities that are based on touch have existed from ancient times. The healing touch and direct person-to-person communication establish relationships that bring healing.

> Parents must be taught how to develop a conscious determination to improve the health and well-being of their 4-A child, along with an expectation of improvement in health and a meaningful, productive life. They need hope—the belief that a desired health goal can be achieved even if it is not a complete cure.

Incidentally, most respondents to surveys indicate that they want physicians to communicate electronically; they want high-tech doctors. But most of all they want more face-to-face time and more personal connections. There should be no reason not to do both. Doctors can facilitate communications and develop relationships through modern technology; even social networks such as Facebook can be used by integrative practitioners to reach an ever-growing number of patients.

Another crucial principle of integrative medicine is communication, coordination, and collaboration between the integrative practitioners themselves, which fosters both supportive relationships and accountability. Dialogue across professional disciplines makes the integrative model work. Here again communication technology offers practitioners an efficient way to connect with one another to better serve patients.

Starting in medical school

The Consortium of Academic Health Centers for Integrative Medicine advocates the training of medical students in integrative care.

They stress the importance of beginning with self-care to enhance a physician's own well-being and to provide a successful example of self-care to his or her patients. A typical school curriculum for the student practitioners includes instruction on how to "walk the walk," how to make the time for healthful personal practices such as proper diet; regular exercise; space for reflection, relaxation, and spirituality; and the importance of relationships and community.

Mind-body medicine skills are often recommended as part of the set of self-care tools. These programs engage the students in an experimental and experiential learning environment, covering disciplines not usually seen in medical schools, such as mindfulness, meditation, diaphragmatic breathing, various relaxation methods, biofeedback, yoga, and tai chi.

One school that has a well-developed program is Monash University Medical School in Australia. Their medical curriculum includes mind-body-based stress reduction as part of a health-enhancement program that is part of an overall self-care plan for students.[3] The three overarching goals at Monash include: (1) student well-being for its own sake; (2) producing holistically minded doctors; and (3) delivering a curriculum that integrates the biomedical, psychological, and social sciences with clinical medicine.

Specific objectives include: (1) the enhancement of personal and professional development by the fostering of positive long-term attitudes and practices with relationship to self-care; (2) laying a foundation for a preventative and holistic approach to medical practice; (3) building important clinical skills that include stress- and lifestyle-management; (4) emphasizing the importance of experimental and hands-on learning; (5) fostering self-directed learning; and (6) advocating integrative learning across disciplines.

In the United States a "healer's art" course has been designed by one of my mentors, Dr. Rachel Naomi Remen, for the medical students at the University of California at San Francisco (UCSF).[4]

The Healer's Art curriculum was designed by Rachel Naomi Remen, M.D., Director of the Institute for the Study of Health and Illness at Commonweal, and Professor of Family and Community Medicine at the University of California, San Francisco (UCSF) School of Medicine. The Healer's Art course was featured in "U.S., News and World Report Best Graduate Schools" issue for the 2002 school year as an example of excellence in medical education. In addition to the UCSF experience, the course has been successfully replicated at 58 medical schools worldwide.[5]

The course is both reflective and process oriented. During the semester a community forms that is perceived as safe for allowing open and honest sharing of experiences, beliefs, and personal truths. Mentoring facilitators participate as equals, and student advisers implement and evaluate the course. It differs radically from other medical school courses in that it employs noncognitive strategies such as imagery, ritual, poetry writing, and journal keeping. Students are taught to discover and nurture their wholeness.

Other topics addressed include grief and loss and the development of compassion. The students are invited to reflect on their feelings of mystery and awe as they experience phenomena that can be observed but not explained. In a final session called "Care of the Soul," they study service as a way of life, exploring the concepts of service, mission, and calling. The student physicians are reminded that a strong belief in the healing benefits of any therapy must accompany any treatments.

Although both of these courses are designed for medical students, many of the concepts are universally applicable to any person who is becoming part of an integrative medical equation, including the parents of 4-A children who may decide to advocate for the adoption of more widespread integrative practices.

The patient corps

What can you as a parent do with this information? You may have already embarked on this journey to find a holistic, integrative physician for your child or children, only to realize as early as day one that there "ain't any out there." While that is not strictly true, in all likelihood it is true in your locality. So what can you do about it?

You can become part of an intentional "patient corps" advocating for change in the medical field. In words attributed to pioneering cultural anthropologist Margaret Mead: "Never doubt that a small group of thoughtful, committed citizens [in this case, patients' parent advocates] can change the world. Indeed, it is the only thing that ever has."

The ultimate objective of a patient corps is to provide the means to form individual integrative-physician-to-pediatric-patient relationships within the corps itself. A more immediate goal is simply to develop a consensus on the collective need to form these relationships. A patient corps is composed of committed parent advocates, all of whom have the same pediatric physician for their children. The leader of a patient corps is usually the individual with the most knowledge and experience with integrative medicine. He or she will start by composing a consensus paper and presenting it to the doctor.

What would such a consensus paper look like? Ideally it would start out with a description of the health crisis in America, demonstrating the enormity of the problem. Then it would go on to express the complementary nature of the principles of holistic, integrative medicine. The presenters want to inform this particular doctor that they have come to the same conclusion collectively: namely that they believe the practice of holistic, integrative medicine will meet all of their children's health care needs. They want to convince the doctor that they value a strong physician-patient relationship. The document serves as an invitation to the doctor to join with them in their quest to learn all they can about integrative medicine and the formation of these relationships. In a polite and diplomatic manner, the patient corps is asking the physician to expand the scope of his practice with implementation of the integrative practice model and to embrace its emphasis on preventative care. "We respect your professional integrity, knowledge, and expertise, and we need someone like you to guide us in assessing a variety of healing modalities. Your triage skills and medical decision making are vital to our quest for healthy family life and personal longevity."

A patient corps would refer their doctor to organizations that have developed comprehensive courses of instruction in holistic, integrative medicine, staffed with prominent leaders, evidence-based research scientists, and clinicians.[6] It is my sincere hope that the efforts of such corps of concerned parents could begin to change the medical climate, for the sake of everyone involved. I strongly recommend that people of influence become leaders in the patient corps movement—employers, administrators, union leaders, clergypersons, corporate executives, school principals and teachers, military commanding officers, leaders of professional associations, insurance executives, and so on.

In the context of the 4-A epidemic, the leaders and members of a patient corps would be parents of children with autism, ADHD, asthma, and allergies. The parents of autistic children in particular have provided for many years a major impetus in the medical advances made in autism therapy. Without their efforts much less would have happened. These parents learned how to work for the healing of their children integratively; they would not settle for waiting the typical twenty years before a particular therapy becomes accepted into clinical medicine. Parent efforts helped give birth to the Defeat Autism Now! (DAN!) movement. The success of the DAN! movement has served as a rallying cry for doctor-patient integrative relationships for 4-A families.

Trends based on sound information and with lasting value turn into movements. Mutual bonds generate communities. Web communities support movements; they organize gatherings, lectures, and conventions, and sell products and services.

Gabriela Mistral, a Nobel Prize–winning Chilean poet, educator, and diplomat, stated it well: "Many things we need can wait. The child cannot. Now is the time his bones are formed, his mind developed. To him we cannot say tomorrow; his name is today."

PARENTING 4-A CHILDREN

Parents are their children's first teachers and primary healers, and I am unaware of any parenting task that is more complex and challenging than that of a 4-A parent/doctor/teacher.

Normal children begin learning at birth from their environment. Sensory information is conveyed to their brains for processing, and the brain cells develop connections and circuitry. But 4-A children do not learn well at all because their toxic brains cannot process the sensory information. What they learn through their five senses gives them a very different sense of the world from that of normal children. Sights and sounds can be distorted. Agreeable tastes and textures can be perceived as unpleasant. Unusual behaviors such as stimming can result from jumbled processing of sensory input on abnormal neuron connections. This abnormality in processing sensory input can result in abnormal fears (visual, auditory, and tactile), colic, picky eating, temper tantrums, and behavioral problems.

Inevitably these children have language development problems that predispose them to more complex learning disorders. The 4-A parent must improve her child's behaviors before intensive learning can begin.

To do this, parents need a lot of support. Parenting stress, depression, and anxiety are always greater for parents of spectrum children than for parents of children with normal development. These parents also report high levels of guilt or self-blame regarding their children's diagnoses of spectrum disorders, especially if they feel that they cannot lay hold of a definitive cause of the disorder. They reflect on things that they did or didn't do during pregnancy or infancy and generally tend to blame themselves for their child's condition.

Mothers of spectrum children feel less satisfied in their parenting role and less competent than parents of children with normal development. This seems to be underscored because these kids have major difficulties forming relationships; they don't look at their parents or show affection, and their parents are unable to calm them when they're angry or upset. The ongoing psychological distress makes mothers feel they are failing to nurture their children well enough. The negative impact on parents raising a spectrum child—less free time, relating to friends and extended family, and the health of their marriage—is often very significant.

This kind of parenting is an intensive-care effort sustained over many years.

The complexities within any spectrum family are too much for one or two people to handle. The job is too big, too demanding. That does not mean that parents are making poor decisions over and over. It means parents have too little support.

Parents need to ask for help by making cooperative arrangements with other spectrum parents, friends, and family. This kind of parenting is an intensive-care effort sustained over many years, and it's challenges will require the thoughtful support of several caring folks, not just one or two parents.

Parents of spectrum children must learn and learn and *learn*. I cannot emphasize enough the value of parenting training, conducted by knowledgeable and skilled mental health counselors who are experienced in all aspects of spectrum challenges. Parents and therapists can collaborate to establish behavioral training for daily functioning at home, and a productive, positive child-parent relationship can be developed. Parents can learn skill sets to help them become proficient at interacting with their children, and they learn how to evaluate education plans and programs in their children's schools.

A very effective teaching program for autistic children was developed in the 1960s, based on behavioral modification principles. It is called applied behavior analysis (ABA), and studies have shown that nearly 50 percent of children who complete the program achieve normal intellectual and educational functioning. In such a program the parents are the principal therapists and the most important people in their child's life.

Parent-child interactions

Dr. Daniel J. Siegel, physician, therapist, parent, researcher, educator and author, believes that infants are born into the world genetically programmed to connect with caregivers and that children who experience a strong attachment early in life do better as they grow up.[7] Studies have found that securely attached children appear to have a number of positive outcomes in their development, including enhanced emotional flexibility, better social functioning, and improved cognitive abilities.

In her book *Your Child's Self-Esteem* Dorothy Briggs writes that every child needs regular "genuine encounters" with his parents, and that a genuine encounter is simply focused attention.[8] This is not just an inherent emotional need. Connecting with adults who love them is an essential factor in the physical development of a child's brain. In other words the growth of the brain is dependent on experiencing a relationship with a caring adult. According to Dr. Siegel, relationships with parents support the development of a child's social, emotional, and cognitive functioning, and how we treat our children makes them who they are. In our communication and connecting, children recognize that their signals have been understood and responded to; they feel nurtured and secure.

Because this is so important to a child's development, parents need to do all they can to normalize their child's ability to connect, first with the parents themselves and then with others.

A parenting program called Hand in Hand in Palo Alto, California, builds on these insights about connecting and security.[9] The teachers and consultants at Hand in Hand have noted how important *emotion* is to the healthy development of a child, along with something they call "listening and limits." Since emotions guide and motivate us, having emotional awareness allows a child to connect with her parents. Parents must help their children understand that they should not fear their emotions, but they cannot let their emotions make decisions for them either. As Julianne Idleman of Hand in Hand says, "All feelings are acceptable even if all behaviors are not."[10] They teach parents how to show comfort and security to a child, even when that child's emotions are out of control, by staying and listening. "Staylistening" enables children to transition through difficult emotional times, assuring them that their wild emotions are OK, while their wild behaviors may not be. The parent stays close to the child, often holding the child until the outburst calms down and ends well—with a warm connection with the parent. This program recommends "time in" rather than "time out" for behavior that needs correction. This way the child can reconnect with the parent rather than being isolated. Patty Wipfler, founder of the Hand in Hand organization, explains that part of the reason spectrum children are in constant, impulsive motion is because they're trying to distract themselves from their tense emotions. They're afraid, deep down, about their ability to survive in this world, fearful about not being OK.

Children need closeness, especially the 4-A child who is trying to relieve emotional stress by crying. Instead of remaining aloof, parents and other caretakers must hold the crying child close, listening to everything and putting up with the struggling, so that the child will learn to equate that with feeling better. This allows that all-important connection to be reestablished. The late Dr. Stanley Greenspan recommended listening through children's tantrums, increasing empathy even while setting limits.[11] Although our natural tendency is to pull away from empathetic closeness when we're involved in angry exchanges, power struggles, or limit setting—because we don't want to appear to empathize with misbehavior—we can learn to empathize with how difficult it is for them to learn new lessons. We can tell our children that we understand how hard it is not to get something, while not caving in to unreasonable demands.

Physical play reinforces the healing process. A spectrum child who is easily distracted needs "playlistening"[12] in the form of roughhousing, pillow fights, wrestling, jumping on the bed, hide-and-seek, and so on. A playful parent is a listening parent, because the parent has adopted a less-powerful role. Maintaining an affectionate tone, the parent plays with lots of bodily contact and cuddling, making eye contact often. Feeling the affection, the child will playfully interact. In playlistening, a parent will follow the child's lead and will keep pursuing the child with affection but will not overwhelm the child, trap the child, or win against the child. Over and over the parent must do whatever makes the child laugh. Laughter heals fear and anxiety. The parent must offer the child survivable challenges. Jumping on the bed, the parent will pretend to be unable to catch the child's feet, giving the child a sense of surviving a threat. Both the parent's patience and the child's laughter will increase the child's confidence and sense of security.

Many times children who have successfully completed long periods of roughhousing play will feel safe enough to show the parent how deeply they really feel by lashing out with a fear-based behavior that must be limited. This is when the parent must move in and physically hold the child close, without any verbal recrimination, sometimes for an hour or more. The child will be furious with the parent and will struggle, but that means that deep fear is coming out. The parent needs to tell the child, "I'll stay until your feelings have subsided." When the feelings have finally run their course, within the safe confines of the parent's loving arms, the child will feel thoroughly relieved.

SUPPORT GROUPS

Needless to say, this kind of parenting is time consuming and energy consuming. To sustain the effort over the long haul, parents must have some outside adult to turn to. Initially parents often receive support from the therapists who work with their children. Support from therapists can significantly help parents' sense of competence and their satisfaction with parenting.

Yet parents often need more. Individual counseling with a mental health clinician can allow an opportunity for the parents to share personal experiences and develop coping strategies that can help them manage their parenting stress. Some kind of self-care is imperative for parents of spectrum children. Often this takes the form of family counseling or marriage counseling. It also takes the form of support groups, either local or online, where parents can relate to other parents of children with similar challenges. Parents might be able to find support groups led by a mental health clinician where they can share information on treatment protocols, behavioral strategies, and self-care. The exchanges with other spectrum parents can provide a sense of community that contrasts with the experience of isolation that is all too common. Support groups are best if they involve face-to-face meetings. As convenient as message boards and online list services may be, real personal contact is the most valuable kind of support.

The financial strain on 4-A families is enormous; so many services are not covered by insurance or provided by schools. Parents may be able to help one another investigate the Medicaid waiver program or Supplemental Security income.

MOVING FORWARD

As health care in America shifts and becomes more expensive, the burden falls more and more on you as 4-A parents to take greater control of your health and that of your children. You will discover if you engage in basic self-care and teach it to your children—exercise, eating more fruits and vegetables, being more mindful, being socially engaged—health care costs will be reduced.

We, like our 4-A kids, are all affected. In this book I have tried to expose you to the valuable insights of my colleagues in order to bring you "up to speed" on a relational level with your integrative pediatrician. Studies continue to emerge in 4-A research, showing for many methods, there is no detectable difference in efficacy when a therapy is administered by parent versus by a professional. We need all hands on deck, and we must continue to impart to one another other as many skills as we can learn. A real partnership between all players is needed as we invent smart ways of sharing ideas and mining data. Our data collection will allow us to learn (a) how the different dimensions (medical, behavioral, educational) relate to one another, (b) which treatments produce which effects on patients with which characteristics, and (c) what the dimensions are of the profound heterogeneity of symptoms.

Learning will occur while we are doing. We know enough already that we do not need to delay. The collaborative model must give rise to further, effective treatment-guided research. I am issuing a call for vigilance, observation, awareness, and detection of the causes and cures of the 4-A epidemic. I have learned to hold tightly to a few key tenets:

- Individuality is primary.
- Mothers are always right.
- Stuff gets in and it cannot get out (toxins, words, and images).
- Children who regain their health prove that nature's strong impulse toward healing overrides genetic structural defects.
- The patient is the best laboratory, as manifested by therapeutic trial.

- The goal is to break the vicious biochemical cycles of inflammation, detoxification, and oxidative stress—and to replace them with a healthy, health-sustaining balance.

BODY, SOUL, AND SPIRIT

Someone once said that the only certain thing in life is change. Change is a constant. Parents who are facing down enduring threats to the health of their children themselves do best when they are able to change. Their children's illness is their signal to change. In this polluted world we need to understand the kids' fight from their perspective, and we need to lend them our perspective. Then we can better help them and ourselves.

> Integrative medicine is premised on patients being treated as whole persons—minds and spirits, as well as physical bodies—who participate actively in their own health.

The way forward involves nurturing a willingness to let go of the past. Often we need to forgive ourselves in order to release ourselves from the past. Forgiveness is a highway to healing. When we cannot flow freely with health, loving life in the present moment, it means we are holding onto the past.

Perceptions, emotions, and attitudes profoundly affect our bodies, for better or for worse. When we make positive changes in the way we are thinking, we can expect healthful changes in our bodies.

Integrative medicine is premised on patients being treated as whole persons—minds and spirits, as well as physical bodies—who participate actively in their own health. One of the most significant and challenging dimensions of integrative medicine is the inclusion of spirituality in both physicians' and patients' (or patient advocates') understanding of health and healing.

Numerous studies have demonstrated the positive effects of prayer, meditation, religious practice, or faith on health outcomes, including the ability to cope with ongoing illness and patients' reported sense of well-being. Increasingly the spirituality of medicine, sometimes called "energy medicine," "mind-body medicine," and "therapeutic touch" has been incorporated into the integrative model.

Spirituality can be defined as the core or inner life, sometimes called the soul but more accurately involving the essence of the human spirit. Since human beings are integrated beings—body, soul (mind and emotions), and spirit—we cannot neglect to weave the spirit into the fabric of healing.

A spiritual perspective in medicine recognizes that the inner life can sustain wounds and illness as well as being a source of vitality and orientation toward healing. All of us, whether we are physicians, parents, or 4-A children, move through changes in our spiritual lives. We all have moments of uncertainty, doubt, sorrow, and suffering. But when there is a mutual willingness to open ourselves to these difficulties and to share them with others, then we have taken the first step toward healing.

For this reason therapies directed toward addressing the functional links between spirit, brain, and body should be particularly effective in treating a range of 4-A symptoms. Many "mind-body therapies" (including hypnosis, mental imagery, biofeedback, progressive muscle relaxation, yoga, meditation, and tai chi) have been found effective for reducing depression, insomnia, anxiety, and acute and chronic pain.

Psychoneuroimmunology is the study of the connection between the mind, emotions, the central nervous system, the autonomic nervous system, and the immune system. This involves the study of the role of the autonomic nervous system, the limbic-hypothalamic-pituitary axis and the neuropeptides and other neuromodulators that self-regulate the immune system. The brain and body communicate with each other through neurons, neuropeptides, and other neurotransmitters. Chemicals in the brain that control our moods, actions, and perceptions are manufactured both by the brain and by the immune system (and other systems). As a result not only do our psychological/emotional states affect the systems of our bodies, but the systems of our bodies also influence our psychological states. A rationale for mind-body regulation is that perception (or imagery) elicits mental and emotional responses, which generate chemical responses in the limbic system, thus activating the pituitary gland and bringing about physiological responses.

Furthermore, evidence is strong for a faith-healing association.[13] Yet significant research is scanty regarding spirituality, the mind-body connection, faith and prayer and the clinical application to the healing of the 4-A population and beyond. Perhaps some of us can explore this further.

Experimental data on prayer or "talking to God" can take many forms, yet a simple attitude of prayerfulness—an all-pervading sense of holiness and a feeling of empathy, caring, and compassion for the entity in need—seems to set the stage for healing. Experiments with people have shown that prayer positively affected headaches, anxiety, and pain. The results of those studies mention enzymes, bacteria, and more, because the prayer had to have influenced the unseen movements inside the body of the person who was being prayed for or with. Remarkably, the affects of prayer do not seem to depend on whether or not the praying person was in the presence of the person being prayed for.

I have learned to include many of our suffering children in my prayers, for I believe that God can touch them. I also include in my prayers their parents, asking God to give them wisdom and trust in dark times and trials. This does not answer all of my questions, but it helps me know what to do next. I cannot determine "what it all means" any more than you can, but I can put my trust in the One who has a purpose for everything.

More than a century ago John Henry Newman summed it up well:

> God knows me and calls me by my name....God has created me to do Him some definite service; He has committed some work to me which He has not committed to another. I have my mission—I never may know it in this life, but I shall be told it in the next.
>
> Somehow I am necessary for His purposes....I have a part in this great work; I am a link in a chain, a bond of connection between persons. He has not created me for naught. I shall do good, I shall do His work; I shall be an angel of peace, a preacher of truth in my own place, while not intending it, if I do but keep His commandments and serve Him in my calling.
>
> Therefore I will trust Him. Whatever, wherever I am, I can never be thrown away. If I am in sickness, my sickness may serve Him; In perplexity, my perplexity may serve Him; If I am in sorrow, my sorrow may serve Him. My sickness, or perplexity, or sorrow may be necessary causes of some great end, which is quite beyond us. He does nothing in vain; He may prolong my life, He may shorten it; He knows what He is about. He may take away my friends, He may throw me among strangers, He may make me feel desolate, make my spirits sink, hide the future from me—still He knows what He is about....
>
> Let me be Thy blind instrument. I ask not to see—I ask not to know—I ask simply to be used.[14]

Appendix A

ADDITIONAL THERAPIES FOR AUTISM

A variety of additional therapies for autism are listed here in alphabetical order, with information about the Autism Treatment Evaluation Checklist (ATEC) at the end of the appendix.

AQUATIC THERAPY

Aquatic therapy can allow parents of spectrum children to help their children manage stress, engage in social encounters, coordinate motor systems, and promote sensory integration. Physical therapists using water therapy report improvements in attention, muscle strength, balance, tolerance of touch, irritability, and maintaining eye contact during their sessions with autistic-ADHD children. The swimming pool provides an excellent environment for spectrum children, who have major difficulty with change and distinguishing relevant from irreverent information. This leads to a particular need for sameness and rituals but leads to problems with sequencing. The simple act of entering the pool from the deck provides children with an opportunity to successfully make a change or a transition. Also, since the pool is a natural place for play, children find it easier to work with others and to tolerate social interaction. In the pool a parent or therapist can use water turbulence and momentum to enhance the child's body awareness. For example, in the game of whirlpool, running water in one direction in a circle is quickly reversed in direction to cause the child to move against the "current." Another example: squirting water with a water gun where body parts are targeted helps desensitize a child and enhance body awareness.

For more information: Aquatic Therapy University (www.aquatictherapy-university.com); Aquatic Integration (www .aquaticintegration.com).

DRAMA THERAPY

Drama is all about relating and developing relationships. Spectrum children crave social connection, and drama therapy facilitates the achievement of those connections. Drama therapy helps children take on and practice new roles as stories are created through actions and rehearsing new behaviors. Drama therapy, role-playing, storytelling, and improvisation (including the use of puppets and masks) help children learn social interaction skills. Some of the benefits of drama therapy are described on pages 124–125 of *Cutting-Edge Therapies for Autism,* by Ken Siri and Tony Lyons (New York: Skyhorse Publishing, 2010): "Drama therapy is effective because it involves action methods, which can be rehearsed or repeated until a skill is learned. An embodied, concrete experience makes skills easier for [spectrum children] to grasp, remember and implement....Neuroscientists looking at the arts, learning, and the brain have discovered that the arts are motivating for children because they create conditions in which attention can be sustained over longer periods of time."

Another benefit from drama therapy is that children receive feedback from other actors, the audience, and one another. Researchers believe that drama strongly engages the mirror neuron system, and because neuroscientists suspect that autism may relate to deficiencies in the mirror neuron system, drama therapy could promote repair of disconnections in the mirror neuron system. Dr. Hans Asperger, who first described Asperger's syndrome in 1944, created an educational program for the boys that he was treating that involved speech therapy, drama, and physical education. (See *Cutting-Edge Therapies for Autism*, page 126.)

To find drama therapists, contact the National Association for Drama Therapy, www.nadt.org.

INTEGRATED PLAY GROUPS

Integrated play groups (IPG) promote socialization, communication, play, and imagination in children on the autism spectrum, while building relationships with typical peers and siblings in natural settings. The IPG model brings together spectrum children in mutually engaging play experiences with more capable peer play partners, guided by a qualified adult facilitator. The IPG programs take place in natural settings including homes, schools, or community sites. Children's individual interests and capabilities influence the structuring of the play sessions. Innately, children are motivated to play, socialize, and form meaningful relationships; the IPG intervention provides the means to bring out the children's developmental potential. The peers are encouraged to be more accepting and responsive of other children who have different ways of playing and communicating. Outcomes for children enrolled in the IPG model show gains in social, communication, and play development, and decreases in isolate and stereotypic play. Of particular interest is a trend that has been observed: skills gained appear to be sustained even after parental support has been withdrawn. The IPG model was created by Pamela Wolfberg, a cofounder of the Autism Institute on Peer Socialization and Play (www.wolfberg.com).

OCCUPATIONAL THERAPY AND SENSORY INTEGRATION

Occupational therapy (OT) uses purposeful activities (occupations) to increase an individual's functional independence. With spectrum kids,

OT can improve their functional fine and gross motor skills; postural control; movement patterns; play skills; social skills; self-help skills; eye-hand coordination; as well as general visual, perceptive, and spatial skills. Occupational therapists who specialize in autism may be skilled in providing sensory integration (SI) therapy as well, which addresses the children's difficulty with processing information through their senses. This can include structured play therapies such as Floortime. (See http://www.icdl.com/dirFloortime/overview/index.shtml.) The late Dr. Anna Jean Ayres, who originally developed SI, defined it as an ability to organize sensory information for use by the many parts of the nervous system in order to work together to promote effective reactions with the environment. For non-autistic children, sensory integration happens naturally, but for ASD kids it's not so easy. Simple tasks such as walking, skipping, swinging, or playing in a park can be overwhelming. These children instinctively try to avoid frightening new experiences, and their ability to acquire new skills is significantly compromised because they cannot properly integrate sensory information (which is why they may rely on self-stimulating or self-regulating behaviors to control their arousal level or to block out perceived adverse stimuli). To a typical spectrum child, sights and sounds in the environment may not make sense; they may seem to be disconnected bits of information. SI brings this information into a meaningful whole. The five sensory systems must be functional and collaborative to facilitate proper sensory integration. Dysfunctional sensory systems and lack of sensory integration can be mistaken for behavioral problems as children try to cope with their deficiencies. Once the sensory issues are corrected, the undesirable behaviors will cease.

For more information about OT, see the fact sheet "Occupational Therapy's Role With Autism," provided by the American Occupational Therapy Association at http://www.aota.org/Consumers/professionals/WhatisOT/RDP/Facts/38517.aspx. For more information about SI, visit the website for the Sensory Motor Integration + Language Enrichment Center (the SMILE Center) at www.smileny.org.

PERSONAL SERVICE CANINES

The results of placing service dogs with spectrum children have been impressive. Children who have been nonverbal for years begin to talk. Stimming behavior and pica (the eating of nonfood items) issues stop completely via the gentle interruption of the dog. Spectrum children whose sensory and anxiety issues make them unable to sit for five minutes are able to sit in a classroom for hours as a result of being tethered to their service dog. Trainers at service dog organizations have developed the skill to know the specific dog that an individual spectrum child needs, and the dogs are trained for the specific needs of the child. Service dogs are with the child around the clock, and the child's family must not allow the dog to become a family pet. Tiffany Denyer, founder and executive director of Wilderwood Service Dogs, explains, "Dogs have an ability to communicate with these children in a way we often don't understand. We know that these dogs allow our clients to have control over something in a world where oftentimes they can't even control the movements of their own bodies." Teachers say that it's good for everyone in their classroom when a child brings his service dog to school. Spectrum children are no longer likely to be shunned, since they now have a dog as a constant companion and the dog loves them unconditionally.

For more information see Wilderwood Service Dogs at www .wilderwood.org.

QIGONG MASSAGE FOR THE AUTISTIC-ADHD CHILD

Qigong massage is a Chinese system adapted for home use by parents of children with mild-to-moderate autism or ADHD. Success with this intervention depends on consistency; a child must receive the fifteen-minute massage daily for at least four months. After diminishing sensory sensitivities, expected benefits include improved eye contact, socialization, and language learning. Trained practitioners administer therapy to children with more severe autism or

ADHD, and Dr. Louisa Silva of the Qigong Sensory Training Institute in Oregon states that "by five months of treatment...autistic behavior decreased by 26 percent; sensory and self-regulation problems decreased by 28 percent."

For more information visit the Qigong Sensory Training Institute website at www.qsti.org.

AUTISM TREATMENT EVALUATION CHECKLIST

The Autism Research Institute has recently provided this research instrument and simple Internet scoring procedure as a valid means of measuring the effectiveness of various treatments for autism.

The Autism Treatment Evaluation Checklist (ATEC) is a one-page, copyright-free form developed by Dr. Bernard Rimland and Dr. Stephen M. Edelson for measuring and evaluating the effectiveness of autism treatments. The test consists of four subtests:

1. Speech/Language/Communication (14 items)

2. Sociability (20 items)

3. Sensory/Cognitive Awareness (18 items)

4. Health/Physical/Behavior (25 items)

Users of the ATEC may have it scored for free (four subscores and a total score) by the Autism Research Institute by entering the responses online on the Autism Treatment Evaluation Checklist Internet Scoring Program at http://www.autism.com/ind_atec.asp.

Appendix B

ADDITIONAL THERAPIES FOR ADHD

A dditional therapies for children with ADHD are listed below in alphabetical order. For information on ADHD therapies and support groups and to find professionals in your locality, go to Children and Adults with ADHD (CHADD) at www.chadd.org/. See "Finding Support." For abstracts from the latest journal articles about alternative therapies for ADHD, go to "Medline Abstracts: Complementary and Alternative Therapies for ADHD" at http://www.medscape.com/viewarticle/438960.

The most effective alternative treatments for ADHD seem to be behavioral in nature. This includes behavior therapy, cognitive behavioral therapy (CBT), parent management training, school-based therapy and classroom management/organization, interpersonal psychotherapy (IPT), working memory therapy, specialized coaching, and support groups.

ADHD COACHING

ADHD coaches are specialized life coaches who have developed techniques based on the cognitive and behavioral distinctives of the various types of ADHD. The coaching works best for older children (including college age) who need help with scheduling, goal setting, confidence building, focusing, general organization, and prioritization and follow-through with tasks. Coaching can take place by telephone if necessary. To be effective, professional coaching must always be added to other therapies.

ART THERAPY

Art therapy (usually in the form of group therapy) is recommended as a means of self-expression and calming for children with ADHD and also for diagnostic purposes. For more about art therapy for children with ADHD, consult the book *Art Therapy and AD/HD* by Diane Stein Safran.

BIOFEEDBACK

With biofeedback (also called neurofeedback) children who are old enough to understand how to participate in the procedures can receive real-time feedback on the patterns of their brainwaves as seen on an EEG, and they can be trained to attain and sustain an EEG pattern that represents an attentive, non-distracted state. The therapy usually involves the equivalent of computer games. All types of ADHD can be addressed, with the most improvement noted for children with inattentive and hyperactive/impulsive types of ADHD. Parents note fewer episodes of oppositional behavior after biofeedback sessions. One significant advantage of biofeedback is that it carries no known side effects. For useful information about a German study that evaluated biofeedback/neurofeedback usage for ADHD children, see Dr. David Rabiner's article entitled "New Study Supports Neurofeedback Treatment for ADHD" posted on SharpBrains (http://www.sharpbrains.com/blog/2009/03/11/new-study-supports-neurofeedback-treatment-for-adhd/).

CRANIOSACRAL FASCIAL THERAPY

Craniosacral fascial therapy (also called simply craniosacral therapy [CST] or cranial sacral therapy/bodywork) is administered by osteopaths, chiropractors, naturopaths, and massage therapists. After a hands-on determination of the "craniosacral rhythm," the therapist gently massages the child's spine and skull, with particular attention to the fascia where the plates of the skull come together. This is thought to restore ease of function to nerves. Besides ADHD, it is used for common stress and pain conditions such as migraines. CST was developed by an osteopath, Dr. William Sutherland, at the end of the nineteenth century.

MASSAGE THERAPY

Basic pediatric massage therapy has been found to improve mood, sense of well-being, and the ability to stay on task for children and adolescents with ADHD.

WORKING MEMORY TRAINING

"Working memory" is the same as short-term memory, and children with ADHD show deficits in this regard—which gives rise to many of their behavioral and social problems. Working memory training usually takes the form of computerized training programs. Results can be inconsistent, depending as they do on many variables, but some children see tangible results.

Appendix C

ADDITIONAL THERAPIES FOR ASTHMA AND ALLERGIES

U p to 50 percent of 4-A children do not respond to conventional treatments for allergies, which are costly and may go on for years; allergy extracts contain preservatives of phenol or glycerin, which many 4-A kids cannot tolerate. In any case allergies to food and other environmental chemicals are not as effectively treated with conventional immunotherapy, although dietary manipulation of foods through elimination diets can benefit many children.

A selection of alternative therapies and treatments for allergies and asthma are listed below in alphabetical order.

ACUPUNCTURE

Acupuncture and acupuncture-based treatments are based on the Chinese theory of meridians, in which needles are inserted into key point of the body. Benefits seem to come from the release of endorphins (the "feel good" chemicals) in the brain, and people with allergies or asthma may attain more relaxed breathing.

BIOFEEDBACK

Biofeedback involves simple electronic devices that help people learn to control involuntary physical responses such as breathing. It can be used to help control asthmatic attacks and stress. Results are mixed, with children and teenagers showing the greatest benefit, according to the Asthma and Allergy Foundation of America.

ENZYME POTENTIATED DESENSITIZATION

Enzyme potentiated desensitization (EPD) differs from allergy shots in three ways: (1) Multiple related antigens are given, whereas allergy shots focus on only a few antigens. (2) EPD doses are much weaker than allergy shots. (3) Given along with allergens is an enzyme, beta glucuronidase, which acts as a catalyst to make the vaccine more potent. The quantities of both the antigen and the beta glucuronidase are smaller than what occur naturally in the body but not as small as in homeopathic treatments. Allergens given in such low doses produce an immunity that eventually leads to desensitization. EPD has not been authorized for use in the United States, although it is available in Canada and the United Kingdom. (Conventional escalating-dose immunotherapy—which is not the same as EPD—has been used to treat tens of millions of people in the United States.)

HOMEOPATHIC DESENSITIZATION

Based on the Law of Similars, diluted homeopathic antigens are ingested to reprogram the immune system to accept the offending substances so that the person's immune system will no longer recognize the antigen as dangerous. Homeopathic resensitization is administered by homeopathic practitioners.

HYPNOTHERAPY

By inducing a hypnotic state in the client, hypnotherapists can make direct suggestions to the person's subconscious mind, engage the client in therapeutic relaxation (helpful for stress-induced asthma), and indicate aversion to certain addictive substances. Hypnotherapy has not been commonly used to treat the allergies and asthma of 4-A children simply because it is rarely used on children in general.

LASER TREATMENT

High-intensity light is used to shrink swollen tissues or unblock sinuses. Considered a temporary solution to allergy-related congestion, it must be administered with care.

MEDICINAL HERBS

Allergy and asthma sufferers sometimes choose various herbal preparations based on their natural antihistamine and anti-inflammatory properties. Care must be exercised in ingesting herbal preparations, however, since the herbs may be in the same botanical family as a substance to which the patient is sensitive. Because of potential aggravation of severe allergies, herbal treatments should be undertaken by your child only in consultation with your integrative pediatrician.

NASAL IRRIGATION

Nasal irrigation is a relatively simple technique for easing nasal congestion and clearing the nasal passageways of allergens. It relies on flushing the nostrils with a purified saline (salt) water solution that is free of contaminants, including iodine (present in iodized salt) and algae (present in some sea salts). It provides temporary relief from allergy symptoms.

RELAXATION TECHNIQUES (INCLUDING MASSAGE, YOGA, AND ART/MUSIC THERAPIES)

To reduce the constriction of airways or inflammation of the skin or other parts of the body that comes from anxiety and stress, various techniques can help to reduce anxiety and allow a child to relax.

SERIAL ENDPOINT TESTING

Holistic integrative practitioners utilize serial endpoint testing (SET) or titration in which responses to specific doses are observed over two to six weeks. A form of intradermal skin testing, SET uses increasing doses of an antigen to determine the concentration at which the reaction changes from negative to positive (which is called the endpoint). Serial endpoint testing is an alternative to other diagnostic tests such as skin prick testing or in vitro testing, and it can be used to determine the antigen dose for immunotherapy. (The endpoint dilution is used as the starting antigen dose.)

Serial endpoint testing can be done for food allergies, especially if a child has difficulties with food elimination diets. Complement antigen testing (to identify immune complex reactions) is a useful diagnostic tool as well. The specific dose antigen is prepared in the physician's office with pure ingredients and no preservatives. The dose of the antigen that is placed in the extract is arrived at though titration and the determination of the strongest dose that does not cause a reaction in the skin. Since nonreactive doses are put into the allergy extract, the desensitization can be done at home by a parent. Benefits can include improved behavior, decreased hyperactivity, improved sleeping habits, and better socialization.

VITAMIN SUPPLEMENTATION

Some of the most popular vitamins and supplements used for allergy/ asthma relief include vitamins A, B_6, B_{12}, C, D, and E; folic acid; quercetin; carotene; magnesium; selenium; and fish oil.

Appendix D

✛ ?! 🫁 ❁

RECOMMENDED RESOURCES

As I stated earlier in this book, the primary intervention for the healing of our 4-A children remains dietary; the appropriate diet of whole foods is fundamental to our treatment plans. To supplement this diet is "to complete"—to complete the nutritional healing program.

There is a unique form of whole foods that is a major component of all the dietary programs I recommend for 4-A children. All of my patients are put on this whole food. It's classified as a whole-food product used to "supplement" or "complete" the diet. This product is Juice Plus.

Hundreds of thousands of phytochemical micronutrients (vitamins, minerals, enzymes) have been identified in fruits and vegetables, and there are many still unknown. The 4-A kids, and all of us, need plenty of whole foods in our diets. A whole food does not contain a large amount of any one nutrient; rather it contains small amounts of numerous nutrients that work together in synergistic balance. By eating whole foods, the synergy is brought into the body. No man-made multinutrient formula can contain all of the vital compounds we need to consume, because metabolically necessary nutrients are yet to be discovered and because it is impossible to re-create nature's synergy in a laboratory. So this bioavailable whole-food concentrate, Juice Plus, is a mainstay of my nutritional therapies. These fruits and vegetables are grown under ideal conditions (mostly organic growing), and the two formulas contain the most nutrient dense fruits and vegetables on the planet. They are juiced immediately after picking, and then they are dried (the powder is more concentrated than the juice itself). The beneficial results in my 4-A patients is astonishing! Juice Plus really works!

It is relatively simple to understand why it works when a review of the clinical research is conducted. It is the most researched neutracentical in the world today. Below are some of the studies conducted on Juice Plus:

- Studies show it delivers key phytonutrients that are absorbed by the body.[1]
- Clinical studies show that Juice Plus helps reduce oxidative stress.[2]
- One clinical study shows it positively impacts markers of chronic inflammation in healthy adults.[3]
- Clinical studies show it helps support a healthy immune system.[4]
- Clinical studies show Juice Plus helps protect DNA.[5]
- Clinical studies show it positively impacts several key indicators of cardiovascular wellness.[6]
- One clinical study shows it supports healthy skin.[7]
- One clinical study shows it supports healthy gums.[8]

For more information on Juice Plus, or to order, visit the Juice Plus website at www.jpcac.com. Or contact Carol Ann Cannizzaro at (407) 869-4363. You can also e-mail her at ccannizzaro@clf.rr.com for more information on Juice Plus, children's health study enrollment, and the hydroponic tower garden.

Appendix E

✜ ?! ❦ ❀

FOR MORE INFORMATION

RECOMMENDED BOOKS AND WEBSITES

Websites

www.healing-autism.com or www.4-AHealing.com (4-A
  Healing Foundation)

www.chadd.org (Children and Adults With ADHD)

www.ewg.org/skindeep/ (For information on allergies
  and sensitivities to cosmetics see the Environmental
  Working Group.)

www.dorisrappmd.com (Doris Rapp, MD, is a leader in the fields of
  environmental medicine and allergies.)

www.aanma.org (Allergy and Asthma Network/Mothers
  of Asthmatics)

www.immune.com/allergy/index.html (Allergy Discussion Group)

www.aafa.org (Asthma and Allergy Foundation of America)

www.add-adhd-help-center.com (Attention Deficit Disorder
  Help Center)

www.gfcfdiet.com/ (The GFCF Diet Intervention-Autism Diet)

www.firstsigns.org (Offers information on early detection/
intervention of autism)

www.autism.org (Global Autism Collaboration)

www.autismndi.com (Autism Network for Dietary Intervention)

www.autism.com (Autism Research Institute and Defeat
Autism Now!)

www.autism-society.org (Autism Society)

www.autismspeaks.org (Autism Speaks)

www.wellnesshealth.com/content.asp?id=343474 (Autism
Suggested Reading)

www.tacanow.org (Talk About Curing Autism—information
and support)

www.unlockingautism.org (Unlocking Autism—information
and support)

www.care2.com/greenliving/make-your-own-non-toxic-cleaning-kit
.html (Care2Make a Difference offers information on how to
make nontoxic cleaning solutions.)

www.foodallergy.org (Food Allergy and Anaphylaxis Network)

www.eatwellguide.org/i.php?pd=Home (Eat Well Guide—markets,
farms, restaurants providing healthy food)

www.godairyfree.org/ (Go Dairy Free offers updated resources
about living with milk allergies, lactose intolerance, gluten-free/
casein-free diets.)

www.familyfoodguide.com/GFCF_diet.html (Visit the Family
Feeding Guide for an overview of the Gluten-Free Casei-
Free Diet.)

www.localharvest.org (Visit Local Harvest to search for local
markets and farms.)

www.ewg.org/foodnews (The Environmental Working Group offers an annual shopper's guide to pesticide-free foods.)

www.pecanbread.com (Pecanbread.com offers information on kids and the specific carbohydrate diet.)

www.aap.org/sections/chim/ParentResources.html (The American Academy of Pediatrics's Section on Complementary and Integrative Medicine offers information and physician listing.)

www.lowoxalate.info/recipes.html (Low Oxalate Diet information and recipes [also GF/CF Diet and SCD])

www.safeminds.org (Offers information about mercury and autism)

www.nutrition-healing.com/index.html (Nutrition Healing provides information on 4-A disorders.)

www.organicconsumers.org/btc/BuyingGuide.cfm (Organic Consumers Association—consumer guide)

www.pesticides.org (Pesticide Education Center—pesticide safety information)

www.beyondpesticides.org/gateway/index.htm (Beyond Pesticides— indexed database of pesticides)

www.nrdc.org/living/labels/ (National Resources Defense Council—product labeling, label lookup and ranking)

www.nsf.org/certified/consumer/listings_main.asp (NSF: The Public Health and Safety Company offers product safety approval, list of NSF-approved products.)

www.ewg.org/tap-water/home (Environmental Working Group— nationwide rankings of city tap water)

www.nrdc.org/water/drinking/qtap.asp (National Resources Defense Council Water offers information about contamination and solutions.)

Books

American Academy of Pediatrics. *ADHD: What Every Parent Needs to Know*. 2nd ed. Grove Village, IL: American Academy of Pediatrics, 2011.

Bock, Kenneth, and Cameron Stauth. *Healing the New Childhood Epidemics: Autism, ADHD, Asthma, and Allergies: The Groundbreaking Program for the 4-A Disorders*. New York: Random House, 2008.

Joneja, Janice Vickerstaff. *Dealing With Food Allergies in Babies and Children*. Boulder, CO: Bull Publishing, 2007.

Nadeau, Kathleen G., Ellen B. Littman, and Patricia O. Quinn. *Understanding Girls with AD/HD*. Silver Spring, MD: Advantage Books, 1999.

Pascal, Cybele. *The Whole Foods Allergy Cookbook: Two Hundred Gourmet and Homestyle Recipes for the Food Allergic Family*. Ridgefield, CT: Vital Health Publishing, 2006.

Rapp, Doris. *Is This Your Child? Discovering and Treating Unrecognized Allergies*. New York: William Morrow, 1991.

Rief, Sandra F. *The ADHD Book of Lists: A Practical Guide for Helping Children and Teens With Attention Deficit Disorder*. San Francisco: Jossey-Bass, 2003.

Rodale, Maria. *Organic Manifesto: How Organic Food Can Heal Our Planet, Feed the World, and Keep Us Safe*. New York: Rodale, 2010.

Magazines

ADDitude: Living Well With Attention Deficit magazine (www .additudemag.com)

Allergic Living: Allergies, Asthma, and Gluten-Free magazine (http:// allergicliving.com/)

Attention: Information and support for people affected by AD/ HD magazine (www.chadd.org/Content/CHADD/ AttentionMagazine/default.htm)

Autism: a bimonthly international journal of research and practice (http://aut.sagepub.com/)

Autism/Asperger's Digest Magazine: real-life information for meeting the real-life challenges of autism spectrum disorders (www .autismdigest.com)

The Autism File: a quarterly journal dealing with all aspects of autism (www.autismfile.com).

Autism Spectrum News: evidence-based news and information (www .mhnews-autism.org)

Autism Spectrum Quarterly: bridging the information gap bridge between the research and general autism communities (www .asquarterly.com)

Coping with Allergies & Asthma magazine (www.copingmag.com/ ana/index.php)

EP/Exceptional Parent: family and professional magazine for the special needs community (www.eparent.com)

HOPELights: monthly activity magazine for children with special needs, including autism (www.hopelightmedia.com)

Living Without: the magazine for people with allergies and food sensitivities (www.livingwithout.com/?s=AF)

GLOSSARY

ADHD: (Attention Deficit Hyperactivity Disorder); a neurobehavioral disorder marked by varying degrees and types of impulsivity, inattentiveness, and/or hyperactivity.

Allergen: Environmental substances that are normally harmless but that provoke a range of symptoms in reactive individuals.

Allergic rhinitis (hay fever): Allergic inflammation of nasal mucous membranes. Here the mast cell release of inflammatory mediators causes patients to suffer from sneezing, runny nose, and watery eyes. Many of these patients will also have asthma, sinusitis, and hives.

Allergy: An exaggerated response of the immune system to specific substances that normally pose no threat to the human body, involving the elevation of specific antibodies due to antigen stimulus.

Analgesic: Pain reliever.

Anaphylaxis: A severe and rapid allergic reaction involving many parts of the body, sometimes fatal.

Anticonvulsant: A drug that decreases abnormal electrical activity within the brain, thus cutting down on the frequency and severity of seizures for someone with a seizure disorder. Sometimes prescribed for people with other disorders.

Antidepressant: One of a number of types of drugs that helps counteract depression by aiding and improving a person's concentration, appetite, sleep, and mood.

Antigen: (From "*anti*body *gen*erator") A cell or molecule that, when introduced into the body, triggers the production of an antibody by the immune system, which will then eliminate the alien and potentially damaging invader. These invaders can be molecules such as pollen or cells such as bacteria.

Antimicrobial: An agent that attacks microscopic organisms such as bacteria, funguses, and viruses.

Antioxidant: A substance that converts free radicals and other reactive oxygen into more stable substances. The primary antioxidant is glutathione; other antioxidants include vitamins A, C, and E.

ASD: autism spectrum disorder

Asthma: A chronic inflammation of the bronchial tubes characterized by symptoms such as wheezing, coughing, chest tightness, and shortness of breath.

Autism: A developmental disorder that encompasses speech development, social development, physical capabilities and tendencies, and cognitive development.

Autism spectrum disorders: Five disorders with distinctive symptoms of autism: (1) autistic disorder, (2) Asperger's syndrome, (3) childhood disintegrative disorder, (4) Rett's disorder, and (5) pervasive developmental disorder—not otherwise specified (PDD-NOS).

Autoimmunity: A misdirected immune response in which the immune system attacks the body's own tissues instead of pathogens.

Beta-agonists (beta-adrenergic drugs): Bronchodilator drugs that, when inhaled into the lungs, relieve asthma symptoms by relaxing the muscles around the bronchial tubes and keeping them relaxed.

Biofilm: A collection of microbes, growing as a community, that form their own matrix in order to adhere together and better communicate with each other. Biofilms can form on a variety of surfaces, but we are referring to the biofilm that forms on the inner surface of the gut. There are two types of biofilm communities: (1) the symbiotic biofilm produced by the good bacteria that protect the gut lining, and (2) pathogenic biofilm, when the bad bacteria gains the upper hand.

Bipolar disorder: A mental disease characterized by cycles of depression and mania.

Blood/brain barrier: Separating the circulating blood from the actual nervous tissue of the brain, the barrier consists of the tightly conjoined endothelial cells that make up the wall of the capillaries, which restrict the passage of fluids (and therefore of toxins) from the blood into the brain itself. Two parts of the brain stem, the area postrema and the nucleus tractus solitarius, lack this protective barrier.

Bronchodilator: A drug that, when inhaled for the relief of an asthma attack, relaxes the constricted bronchial muscles and thereby causes the bronchial tubes to widen. Short-acting bronchodilators help during asthma attacks, and long-acting types need to be taken daily, often with a steroid.

Bronchospasm: A term descriptive of asthma, namely a constriction of the muscles of the bronchial walls that causes labored breathing, wheezing, and other symptoms. Children and adults with asthma can develop broncho-spasm symptoms when they get exposed to any one of a number of triggers (e.g., exercise, especially in cool weather outdoors; a virus; an allergen; or an irritant).

Candida albicans: A yeastlike fungus that can infect the mouth, intestines, vagina, and surrounding skin. It normally maintains a small presence in the intestines, where it is not harmful. An overgrowth can lead to candidiasis.

Candidiasis (oral): Commonly known as "thrush," yeast overgrowth, or yeast infection, candidiasis indicates that the opportunistic *Candida albicans* fungus has caused white spots on the tongue and inside of the mouth.

Candidiasis (gut): Causing gut dysbiosis through the same process causing gut inflammation.

Carbohydrates: Mainly sugars and starches, sources of calories (energy) that come in simple forms (sugars) and complex forms (starches and fiber), which are broken down in the body into the simple sugar glucose. Carbohydrates are classified into mono-, di-, tri-, poly-, and heterosaccharides. The most basic and smallest carbohydrates are the monosaccharides.

Casein: The most common protein found in milk.

Casomorphine: A product of the digestion of casein (from dairy products), a peptide that is known as an opioid because it shares a chemical structure based on morphine.

Chelation therapy: Chelation therapy removes heavy metals (most commonly mercury, lead, and arsenic) from the body through the administration of che-lating agents (frequently dimercaptosuccinic acid, or DMSA). A chelating agent makes chemical bonds with metal ions, resulting in a water-soluble com-plex that enters the bloodstream and gets excreted through normal processes.

Commonality: A shared set of attributes or features. In the context of this book, the word refers to an aggregate of environmental conditions and influences that have caused the epidemic of 4-A disorders.

Comorbid: The dual (or more) occurrence of medical conditions in the same person, for example, co-occurring 4-A diagnoses and frequent inflammations and infections.

Corticosteroids: Anti-inflammatory drugs taken daily for long-term prevention of asthma attacks.

Cytokines: Regulatory proteins produced by the immune system to facilitate communication and interactions between cells.

Detoxication: Neutralization and elimination of internal toxins derived from normal metabolic processes in the body.

Detoxification: Neutralization and elimination of external toxins that have gained entry into the body.

Disaccharides: A class of sugars (including sucrose and lactose) that yield two monosaccharide molecules.

DMSA (dimercaptosuccinic acid): One of several chelating agents that make chemical bonds with metal ions, resulting in a water-soluble complex that enters the bloodstream and gets excreted through normal body processes.

Dopamine: A brain chemical (neurotransmitter) associated with feelings of pleasure as well as with movement, emotion, and motivation. Low dopamine levels are predictable with attention deficit disorder and autism.

Dysbiosis: The condition that results when the natural balance of bacterial flora in the GI tract is disturbed, with a number of possible symptoms including diarrhea, nutritional deficits, and discomfort.

Echolalia: Repetition of another person's words.

Eczema (atopic dermatitis): Allergic inflammation of the skin, often beginning in infancy, appearing after a baby stops breast feeding. This skin has a raised red eruption that forms scaling crusts with itching as a principle symptom. Eczema has a familial occurrence with long histories of allergies, asthma, and hay fever.

Enterocytes: Specialized cells in the small intestine that absorb nutrients, electrolytes, and water

Eosinophils: Are a type of white blood cell, part of the immune system, that contain particles filled with chemicals to conquer infections. The blood does not carry a large number of eosinophils unless your body needs to produce more of them in an allergic or inflammatory response, or in the case of parasitic infections.

Free radical: (Short for "oxygen-free radical") An unstable substance with an unpaired electron that causes random damage to nearby molecules of the body as it reacts with them in an effort to "steal" the missing electron.

GABA: Gamma-aminobutyric acid, a neurotransmitter that helps the brain maintain muscle control and mood.

Glutamate: An amino acid (a building block for proteins) and a neurotransmitter in the central nervous system.

Glutathione: An antioxidant, often with a low activity level in 4-A children.

Gluten: A protein with sticky qualities that comes from the outer endosperm of wheat seeds and related grains.

Gluteomorphine: A product of the digestion of gluten (from grains), a peptide that is known as an opioid because it shares a chemical structure based on morphine.

Histamine: Substance released by mast cells when an allergen is encountered. Histamine increases the permeability of blood vessel walls and causes itching, hives, eye irritation, and sneezing in the person having the allergic reaction.

Hyperglycemia: High blood sugar. Symptoms include hyperactivity and self-stimulation in spectrum children.

Hyperlexia: Repetitive speech.

Hypoglycemia: Low blood sugar. Symptoms include disorientation, headache, verbal difficulty, shakiness, anxiety (and tantrums in children), and fatigue.

IgA (immunoglobulin A): Produced by gut wall lymphocytes to kill invading bacteria, funguses, viruses, and parasites, thus protecting the gut wall epithelium. Unhealthy gut flora leads to a reduction in the number of gut wall cells producing IgA, which means less protection from damage from the toxic environment.

IgE (immunoglobulin E): Produced by plasma cells and lymphocytes, a protein that works by binding to allergens. It triggers the release of chemicals that can cause inflammation (i.e., an "allergic reaction").

IgG (immunoglobulin G): A protein produced by plasma cells and lymphocytes, also known as gamma globulin. A major class of immunoglobulins that includes many of the antibodies that circulate in the blood.

IgM (immunoglobulin M): An immunoglobulin that supplies "first-responder" antibodies that are replaced by other antibodies later in the immune response.

Immune system: A self-defense system designed to protect the human body from harmful invasion from the outside. The complete immune response involves many organs and types of tissue or cells, including the thymus; the spleen; the lymph nodes; lymphoid tissue found in special deposits throughout the body; lymphocytes (white blood cells), including T cells; and antibodies.

Inflammation: The immune system's protective response, elicited by injury, damage, or destruction of tissues. Inflammation serves to wall off the damaged tissue so that the injurious agent can be sequestered, diluted, and eliminated.

Integrative medicine: Relationships-centered care (doctor-patient) in which the doctor seeks to understand not only the biological aspect of health but also the patient's culture, beliefs, and unique characteristics and in which the patient is regarded as an active partner in attaining and maintaining health through attention to lifestyle choices as well as medical interventions. As defined by the American College for the Advancement of Medicine (http://www.acamnet.org): *Integrative medicine combines conventional care with alternative medicine to improve patient care. Rather than practice one type of medicine, integrative physicians will often combine therapies and treatment approaches to ensure the best results for their patients.*

Interferon: A protein that boosts immune protection by interfering with the growth of viruses and other intracellular invaders.

Interleukin: One of a group of cytokines (secreted proteins/signaling molecules) that help regulate cell-mediated immunity.

Intolerance: A reaction to food that does not involve the immune system. An intolerance presupposes the absence of a particular chemical or physiologic process needed to digest a food substance. For example, the lack of a digestive enzyme may result in a food intolerance.

Macrophages: Large white blood cells that help the body fight off infections by ingesting the disease-causing organism. Macrophages are "big eaters," named from the Greek from *makros* ("large") and *phagein* ("eat").

Mast cells: Cells in connective tissue that release histamine and other inflammatory chemicals when injured in an allergic reaction.

Melatonin: A hormone that helps control the sleep cycle as well as other functions.

Metabolic dysfunction: A compromised biochemical process within the human body.

Metabolism: The chemical and physical processes of a human body that convert and use food, water, air, light, and other nutrients.

Methylation: A metabolic pathway that is part of the normal detoxification system of the body in which molecules for detoxification and antioxidation are produced.

Methylphenidate: The most common class of ADHD drugs (includes Ritalin). The effects of methylphenidates are similar to those of amphetamines, only milder, and they can help calm children with ADHD.

Microbiome: The totality of the microflora (whether beneficial, opportunistic, or transitional) in a person's gut.

Monosaccharides: Simple sugars, including glucose, fructose, and galactose, that cannot be broken down further into other sugars.

Motor tic: A repeated twitching of a group of muscles, either simple such as eye-blinking or complex such as twirling in place. Vocal tics involve the muscles that produce speech. Tics arise from the part of the brain that controls automatic movements and impulsivity.

Neuropsychiatric symptomatology: The cognitive and behavioral symptoms of a disorder that include both psychic and organic aspects.

Neurotoxin: A substance that blocks nerve signals.

Neurotransmitter: A chemical released from a nerve cell to transmit a message to another nerve, muscle, organ, or some other body tissue.

Neutrophils: The type of white blood cells found in abundance in the bloodstream that serve as "first responders" when an inflammation occurs. Neutrophils are filled with enzymes that help them kill and digest harmful microorganisms. They predominate in pus, giving it its yellowish-white color.

Oxidative stress: The overabundance of oxygen-free radicals in the body, which lead to cell and tissue damage.

Pathogen: A microorganism that causes a disease (i.e., a bacterium or a virus).

Pathogenic: The capability of causing disease.

Pathologic, pathological: Diseased.

Pathophysiology: The study of the abnormalities of body function that characterize particular diseases or syndromes.

Prebiotics: Foods that promote the growth of beneficial bacteria: legumes, peas, soy beans, garlic, onion, leeks, and chives.

Probiotics: Foods and supplements that contain live "good bacteria" similar to those found in a healthy human gut.

Psychoactive: Affecting a person's mind. The word is used mostly to refer to drugs.

Sensitivity: Any adverse reaction in the body that comes from exposure to a sensitizing agent in the environment. A sensitivity can involve antibodies and other immune processes. Food and chemical reactions are sensitivities.

Serotonin: 5-hydroxytryptamine, a neurotransmitting hormone that transmits nerve signals between nerve cells, causes blood vessels to narrow, and affects a person's level of contentment.

Sinusitis: Allergic inflammation of sinus cavities; sinus infection.

Status asthmaticus: A serious condition in which asthma attacks follow quickly after one another without a gap.

Stimming: short for "self-stimulation," repetitive body movements such as rocking, hand-flapping, or spinning that stimulate or distract the child from internal discomforts.

Stimulant: A drug that works by increasing dopamine levels in the brain. Dosages increase gradually (so as to avoid "hyper" behavior or addiction) until the desired therapeutic effect has been reached.

Systems medicine: A study of the functional biologic systems of the body. The inevitable conclusion of systems medicine is that everything is related.

T cells: White blood cells also known as lymphocytes that play an important role in the immune response of the human body. The *T* stands for *thymus*, the gland in which the cells reach maturity and from which they are released.

Th-1 cells: Cells that can attack pathogens directly, or stimulate other immune cells to attack, in a response known as cell-mediated immunity because it is performed by the cells themselves.

Th-2 cells: Cells that attack pathogens by sending messages to encourage other immune cells to produce antibodies, which in turn attack pathogens such as bacteria, viruses, and allergens. These cells do not enter cells that have been attacked by pathogen, as Th-1 cells do.

Theophylline: A type of bronchodilator drug that can help control mild asthma, especially at night.

Urticaria (hives): Occurs in the skin as welts. Lesions appear swollen, raised, and red with different sizes and shapes. The skin allows us to actually see the results of inflammatory mediators at work.

Vasoactive: Causing dilation or constriction of the blood vessels.

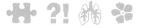

NOTES

CHAPTER 1: FOUR NEW CHILDHOOD EPIDEMICS

1. Maria Rodale, *Organic Manifesto* (New York: Rodale, 2010), 18. Original endnotes within quote: *Centers for Disease Control and Prevention, "Autism Spectrum Disorders (ASDs)," http://www .cdc.gov/ncbddd/autism/ data.html (accessed December 7, 2011). **Liz Szabo, "Food Allergies in Kids Soar," *USA Today*, October 23, 2008, 70.

CHAPTER 2: WHAT'S TO BLAME FOR THE 4-A EPIDEMIC?

1. Rodale, *Organic Manifesto*, 12–13. Original endnote within quote: *United States Geological Survey, "Water Science for Schools: Irrigation Water Use," http://ga.water.usgs.gov/edu/wuir.html (accessed December 7, 2011).

2. Kenneth Bock and Cameron Stauth, *Healing the New Childhood Epidemics: Autism, ADHD, Asthma, and Allergies* (New York: Ballantine Books, 2007), 20–21.

3. Ibid., 123.

4. Ibid., no page given.

5. Ibid.

6. Bruno Bettelheim, *The Empty Fortress: Infantile Autism and the Birth of the Self* (New York: The Free Press, 1967).

7.   Bernard Rimland, *Infantile Autism: The Syndrome and Its Implications for a Neural Theory of Behavior* (New York: Prentice-Hall, 1964). See also the website for the Autism Research Institute at http://www.autism .com/.

CHAPTER 3: WHY THE INTEGRATIVE APPROACH IS DIFFERENT—AND BETTER

1.   For more recommendations and information, read the article "Clinician Registry," http://autism.com/pro_danlists_results .asp?list=US&type=1 (accessed December 7, 2011).

2.   American College for the Advancement of Medicine, "What Is Integrative Medicine?," http://www.acamnet.org/site/c .ltJWJ4MPIwE/ b.5457445/k.CCC8/What_is_Integrative_Medicine.htm (accessed December 7, 2011).

3.   See Glossary for definitions of many of these terms, some of which we will discuss in depth in the chapters of this book.

4.   PANDAS is an abbreviation for Pediatric Autoimmune Neuropsychiatric Disorders Associated with Streptococcal Infections, sometimes helpful to diagnose in situations in which children have had infections such as strep throat and scarlet fever, subsequent to which they rapidly developed a tic disorder or obsessive-compulsive disorder. It is surmised that the infection sets up an autoimmune reaction.

5.   ASO stands for Antistreptolysin O. The titer (blood test) measures antibodies against streptolysin O, a substance produced by group A Streptococcus bacteria.

6.   Another blood test to measure antibodies against group A Streptococcus bacteria.

CHAPTER 4: AUTISM

1.   For an excellent overview of autism, go to the website of the Autism Research Institute at http://www.autism.com/fam_autism_overview.asp.

2.   Autism Research Institute http://www.autism.com/index_b.asp.

3.   Stephen Edelson, "The 'Medically Fragile' Subtype: Documenting 32 Children," *Autism Research Review International*, 23, no. 3 (December 2009): 3.

4.   Ibid.

5.   See a more complete chart in Stephanie Cave, *What Your Doctor May Not Tell You About Children's Vaccinations* (New York: Warner, 2001), 63–64, which has been adapted by Dr. Cave from a research paper, "Autism: A Unique Type of Mercury Poisoning," by Sallie Bernard and associates, copyright ARC Research, 14 Commerce Dr., Cranford, NJ 07016, April 21, 2000.

6.   Dr. Don Colbert and I have included interesting data on this subject in our book, *Eat This and Live! for Kids.*

7.   Nutrition Healing, "Low Oxalate Diet," http://www.nutrition -healing.com/lowoxalate.html (accessed December 13, 2011).

CHAPTER 5: ADHD
(ATTENTION DEFICIT HYPERACTIVITY DISORDER)

1.   The name "Ring of Fire" is derived from the appearance of the brain scan, which shows a ring of hyperactivity in the prefrontal cortex, both parietal lobes, and the anterior cingulate gyrus.

2.   Daniel G. Amen, *Healing ADD* (New York: Berkley/Penguin Putnam, 2001).

CHAPTER 6: THE ASTHMA EPIDEMIC

1.   From American Lung Association. Epidemiology & Statistics Unit, Research and Program Services, Trends in Asthma Morbidity and Mortality, November 2007, as referenced in American Academy of Allergy and Asthma Immunology, "Asthma Statistics," http://www.aaaai.org/about-the-aaaai/ newsroom/asthma-statistics.aspx (accessed December 13, 2011).

2.   Centers for Disease Control, "Surveillance for Asthma—United States, 1960–1995," MMWR Surveillance Summaries, April 24,1998; 47 (SS-1) http://www.cdc.gov/mmwr/preview/mmwrhtml/00052262.htm (accessed December 16, 2011).

3.   Centers for Disease Control and Prevention, "Asthma in the U.S.: Growing Every Year," *Vital Signs,* May 2011.

4.   Bock and Stauth, *Healing the New Childhood Epidemics,* 124.

5.   Ibid.

6.   Asthma and Allergy Foundation of America, "Alternative Therapies," http://www.aafa.org/display.cfm?id=9&sub=19&cont=254 (accessed December 13, 2011).

CHAPTER 7: ALLERGIES—THE UNIVERSAL THREAT

1.   Compiled from text by Doris Rapp, *Is This Your Child? Discovering and Treating Unrecognized Allergies* (New York: William Morrow, 1991), 65–83.

2.   N. Campbell-McBride, "Gut and Psychology Syndrome (GAP Syndrome or GAPS)," http://mindd.org/serendipity/uploads/pdf/Campbell-McBrideGAPSArticle-MinddFoundation.pdf (accessed December 13, 2011). See also Dr. Campbell-McBride's website, www .doctor-natasha.com (accessed December 13, 2011).

CHAPTER 9: HEALING THROUGH NUTRITIONAL THERAPY

1.   Enzyme Stuff, "Harvard Clinic Scientist Finds Gut and Autism Link," http://www.enzymestuff.com/rtgutresearch.htm (accessed December 13, 2011).

2.   "Treatments for Autism Spectrum Disorder Through Special Diets: Changing a Diet Can Transform a Life," *Living Without* magazine, as referenced on The Autism File, http://www.autismfile.com/diet-nutrition/treatments-for-autism-spectrum-disorder-through-special-diets (accessed December 13, 2011).

3.   Such lists are not difficult to find in diet literature and on the Internet. See Appendix E, "For More Information," for some suggestions.

4.   Modified from Rapp, *Is This Your Child?*, 166–167.

5.   Based on Doris Rapp, "If You Suspect Food and Environmental Allergies," February 8, 2010, http://www.drrapp.com/2010/02/18/treatment-if-you-suspect-food-environmental-allergies-free-report/ (accessed February 7, 2012).

6.   An excellent starting place is the website www.pecanbread.com.

7.   See a list of legal/illegal foods on the SCD compiled by Kim Hesche: http://www.pecanbread.com/p/legal_illegal_a-c.htm (accessed December 14, 2011).

8.   Jon Pangborn and Sidney Baker, *Autism: Effective Biomedical Treatments* (San Diego: Autism Research Institute, 2005).

9.   Nutrition Healing, "Low Oxalate Diet," http://www.nutrition-healing.com/lowoxalate.html (accessed December 14, 2011).

10. A complete list of high oxalate foods is available on the University of Pennsylvania Medical Center website, www.upmc.com/HealthAtoZ/ patienteducation/U/Pages/lowoxalatediet.aspx (accessed December 14, 2011) and at www.lowoxalate.info/food_ lists/alph_oxstat_chart .pdf (accessed December 14, 2011).

CHAPTER 10: HEALING THROUGH SUPPLEMENTATION THERAPY

1   Bock and Stauth, *Healing the New Childhood Epidemics*, 248.

2. From a personal e-mail to the author.

3. A summary of research results for essential oils (not directed specifically to 4-A children) can be found in the article "Aromatherapy: Current and Emerging Applications" by Sala Horowitz, PhD, in the journal *Alternative and Complementary Therapies*, 17, no. 1 (February 2011): 28, published by Mary Ann Liebert, Inc. [liebertpub.com]. The table has been derived from two other recommended resources: Carol Schiller and David Schiller, *The Aromatherapy Encyclopedia: A Concise Guide to Over 385 Plant Oils* (Laguna Beach, CA.: Basic Health Publications, Inc., 2008); and Sue Clarke, *Essential Chemistry for Aromatherapy*, 2d ed. (Edinburgh: Churchill Livingstone, 2008). I also recommend David Stewart, *Healing Oils of the Bible* (Marble Hill, MO: Care Publications, 2004), the website www .raindroptraining.com, and the website www .drfriedmannessentialoils.com for information about oils that have helped 4-A children.

4. This supplement was developed by Dr. T. C. Theoharides. See http://www.algonot.com/neuroprotek.php (accessed December 14, 2011).

CHAPTER 11: HEALING THROUGH DETOXIFICATION THERAPY

1. Alejandro Junger, *Clean: The Revolutionary Program to Restore the Body's Natural Ability to Heal Itself* (New York: HarperCollins, 2009), 9.

2. Alejandro Junger, "The Clean Program At-a-Glance Chart," http:// www .cleanprogram.com/files/clean-planner.pdf (accessed December 14, 2011).

3. Rapp, *Is This Your Child?*, 260–261.

CHAPTER 12: HEALING THROUGH MEDICATION

1. Bock and Stauth, *Healing the New Childhood Epidemics*, 340.

CONCLUSION: EMPOWERING PARENTS

1. See statement of the Consortium of Academic Health Centers for Integrative Medicine at http://www.imconsortium.org/about/home.html (accessed December 14, 2011).

2. K. B. Thomas, "General Practice Consultations: Is There Any Point in Being Positive?," *British Medical Journal* 294 (May 9, 1987): 1200–1202, http://www.ncbi.nlm.nih.gov/pmc/articles/PMC1246362/pdf/bmjcred00019-0024.pdf (accessed December 14, 2011).

3. Craig Hassed, Victor S. Sierpina, and Mary Jo Kreitzer, "The Health Enhancement Program at Monash University Medical School," *The Journal of Science and Healing* 4 (November 2008): 394–397.

4. Jennifer Pearson, "Teaching the Art of Healing," *Minnesota Medicine*, April 2009, http://www.ishiprograms.org/wp-content/uploads/09_MN-Med_Teaching-Art-of-Healing___Pearson.pdf (accessed December 14, 2011).

5. Quote is from Creighton University School of Medicine (Omaha, Nebraska, and Phoenix, Arizona) description of course offerings at http://medschool.creighton.edu/medicine/admin/ome/thehealersart/index.php (accessed December 14, 2011).

6. Three prominent organizations are the American College for Advancement in Medicine (www.acamnet.org), the American Holistic Medical Association (www.holisticmedicine.org), and the Institute for Functional Medicine (www.functionalmedicine.org). For continuing self-education, you could consult resources such as the *Well Being Journal* (www.wellbeingjournal.com).

7. I recommend Dr. Siegel's books, including *Parenting From the Inside Out* (New York: Jeremy P. Tarcher/Penguin, 2004), and *The Whole-Brain Child: 12 Revolutionary Strategies to Nurture Your Child's Developing Mind, Survive Everyday Parenting Struggles, and Help Your Family Thrive* (New York: Delacorte/Random House, 2011). See also "Attachment and Self-Understanding: Parenting With the Brain in Mind," a journal article that became a chapter in *Parenting From the Inside Out*, viewable at http://www.attach.org/AttachmentandSelf-understanding1.pdf (accessed December 15, 2011).

8. Dorothy Corkille Briggs, *Your Child's Self-Esteem* (New York: Broadway Books/Random House, 1970).

9. Hand in Hand: Nurturing the Parent-Child Connection, www.handinhandparenting.org/ (accessed December 15, 2011).

10. Julianne Idleman, "Parent Education: Dealing With Emotions," http://www.handinhandparenting.org/news/173/64/Parent-Science -101---Part-Two-Emotion (accessed December 15, 2011)

11. Stanley I. Greenspan, *The Secure Child: Helping Our Children Feel Safe and Confident in a Changing World* (Cambridge, MA: De Capo Press/ Perseus Books, 2002).

12. "Playlistening" is the term used by the Hand in Hand program.

13. To cite a lengthy but partial list of books and articles that explore this association, see the following: Deidre Davis Brigham, *Imagery for Getting Well: Clinical Applications of Behavioral Medicine* (New York: W. W. Norton, 1996); Larry Dossey, *Healing Words: The Power of Prayer and the Practice of Medicine* (New York: HarperCollins, 1993); E. Ernst, M. H. Pittler, B. Wider, and K. Boddy, "Mind-Body Therapies: Are the Trial Data Getting Stronger?" *Alternative Therapies In Health and Medicine* 13 (September/October 2007): 62–64; Sala Horowitz, "Effect of Positive Emotions on Health: Hope and Humor," *Alternative and Complementary Therapies* 15 (August 2009): 196–202; Dharma Singh Khalsa and Cameron Stauth, *Meditation as Medicine: Activate the Power of Your Natural Healing Force* (New York: Fireside2001); Jeff Levin, "How Faith Heals: A Theoretical Model," *Explore: The Journal of Science and Healing* 5 (March 2009): 77–96.

14. John Henry Cardinal Newman, *Meditations and Devotions*, "Meditations on Christian Doctrine" (New York: Longmans, Green, & Co., 1893), 400–402.

APPENDIX D: RECOMMENDED RESOURCES

1. *Molecular Nutrition and Food Research* 54 (2010): 1506–1514; *Asia Pacific Journal of Clinical Nutrition* 16 (2007): 411–421; *Journal of Nutrition* 136 (2006): 2606–2610; *eCAM* 4 (2007): 455–462; *Journal of American College of Nutrition* 23 (2004): 205–211; *Journal of Nutrition* 133 (2003): 2188–2193; *Journal of Human Nutrition and Dietetics* 13 (2000): 21–27; *Nutrition Research* 19 (1999): 1507–1518; *Integrative Medicine* 2 (1999): 3–10; *Current Therapeutic Research* 57 (1996): 445–461; *International Journal of Food Sciences and Nutrition* 60 (2009): S65–75; *Clinical Chemistry and Laboratory Medicine* 44 (2006): 391–395; *Skin Pharmacology and Physiology* 25 (2012):2–8, epub ahead of print.

2. *Molecular Nutrition and Food Research* 54 (2010): 1506–1514; *Asia Pacific Journal of Clinical Nutrition* 16 (2007): 411–421; *Journal of Nutrition* 136 (2006): 2606–2610; *Journal of Human Nutrition and Dietetics* 13 (2000): 21–27; *Current Therapeutic Research* 57 (1996): 445–461; *Journal of Nutrition* 137 (2007): 2737–2741; *Medicine & Science in Sports & Exercise* 41 (2009): 155–163; *Medicine & Science in Sports & Exercise* 38 (2006): 1098–1105; *Medicine & Science in Sports & Exercise* 43 (2011): 501–508; *Journal of the American College of Nutrition* 30, no. 1 (2011): 49–56; *Clinical Chemistry and Laboratory Medicine* 44 (2006): 391–395.

3. *Molecular Nutrition and Food Research* 54 (2010): 1506–1514; *Journal of Nutrition* 137 (2007): 2737–2741.

4. *Journal of Nutrition* 136 (2006): 2606–2610; *Integrative Medicine* 2 (1999): 3–10; *Journal of Nutrition* 137 (2007): 2737–2741; *British Journal of Nutrition* 105 (2011): 118–122.

5. *Journal of Nutrition* 136 (2006): 2606–2610; *Nutrition Research* 19 (1999): 1507–1518.

6. *Asia Pacific Journal of Clinical Nutrition* 16 (2007): 411–421; *eCAM* 4 (2007): 455–462; *Journal of Nutrition* 133 (2003): 2188–2193; *Nutrition Research* 23 (2003): 1221–1228; *Journal of the American College of Cardiology* 41 (2003): 1744–1749; *Journal of the American College of Nutrition* 30, no. 1 (2011): 49–56; *Skin Pharmacology and Physiology* 25 (2012): 2–8, epub ahead of print.

7. *Skin Pharmacology and Physiology* 25 (2012): 2–8, epub ahead of print.

8. *Journal of Clinical Peridontology* 2011, epub ahead of print.

INDEX

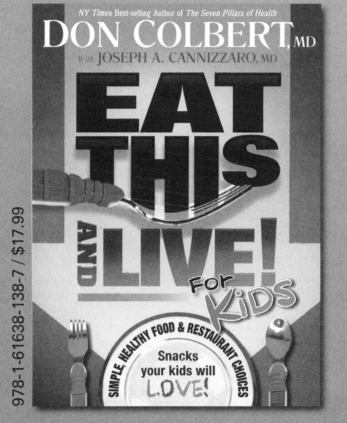
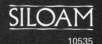